PENGUIN BOOKS

CALM FOR LIFE

Paul Wilson thrives in several high-stress worlds: successful businessman, strategic consultant to major corporations, father to a teenager and two young children, and director of a hospital and medical research foundation.

To thrive in these worlds, he has mastered the secrets of calm. His first book, *The Calm Technique*, is widely acknowledged as one of the most influential books in the genre. His second, *The Big Book of Calm*, has been translated into twenty languages. His third, *The Little Book of Calm*, has spent more than two years at the top of the best-seller lists, with sales of over three million copies. The success continues with *Calm at Work* and *The Little Book of Calm at Work*.

You can contact the author at www.calmcentre.com

If you would like to know how calm can transform your workplace, go to www.calmatwork.com

Calm
for Life

The relaxed way to take control of your life,
health, fortune and peace of mind

Paul Wilson

PENGUIN BOOKS

PENGUIN BOOKS

Published by the Penguin Group
Penguin Books Ltd, 27 Wrights Lane, London W8 5TZ, England
Penguin Putnam Inc., 375 Hudson Street, New York, New York 10014, USA
Penguin Books Australia Ltd, Ringwood, Victoria, Australia
Penguin Books Canada Ltd, 10 Alcorn Avenue, Toronto, Ontario, Canada M4V 3B2
Penguin Books (NZ) Ltd, Private Bag 102902, NSMC, Auckland, New Zealand

Penguin Books Ltd, Registered Offices: Harmondsworth, Middlesex, England

First published by Penguin Books Australia Ltd 2000
Published in Great Britain in Penguin Books 2000

1 3 5 7 9 10 8 6 4 2

The information contained in this book (and any accompanying printed or electronically
published material) has been carefully researched and compiled, but is not intended to
replace the attention or advice of a physician or other healthcare professional. Neither the
author nor the publisher will be held responsible or liable for any action or claim
howsoever arising or resulting from the use of this book or any information contained in
it. If you wish to embark on any dietary, drug, exercise or other lifestyle change intended
to prevent or treat a specific disease or condition, you should first consult with and seek
medical advice from a qualified healthcare professional.

Set in Bembo
Printed in England by Clays Ltd, St Ives plc

Calm for Life is dedicated to all those who have joined
or are about to join me on the mission to spread calm.

Where do I start? To the contributors to the Calm Centre –
the therapists, researchers, academics, spiritual advisors, artists,
programmers and musicians who give so generously of their time.
To those who have openly shared their personal experiences
and learning with us in the preparation of this book.
To the selfless supporters of the charities we are aligned with.
And to all those who recognise there is as much to celebrate and
feel good about in today's world as there is to condemn.

CONTENTS

A NOTE FROM PAUL WILSON   ix

INTRODUCTION
WHAT WILL IT TAKE?   1

1
THE AGE OF CALM   9

The spread of calm   11
The benefits of calm   16

2
THE WORLD'S MOST
POWERFUL INDIVIDUAL   37

3
AN IRON WILL AND A
STEEL-TRAP MIND   55

The centre of the whole   57
The whole   71
The centre   81

4
THE CALM CENTRE'S NINE
MENTAL POWERS   97

5
CALM FROM THE CENTRE   109

6
A FEW STEPS, MANY PATHS   127

Step 1   129
Step 2   130
Step 3   145
Step 4   176

7
FROM CALM COMES POWER   181

8
APPLICATIONS OF DEEP CALM   245

Calm for wellness and longevity   247
Calm for success and prosperity   291
Calm and be happy   301
Calm relationships   306
A calm change of habit   312
The spiritual side to calm   314
The big picture   328
Calm major, calm minor   331

9
CALM FOR THE REST
OF YOUR LIFE   333

INDEX   345

A NOTE FROM PAUL WILSON

By the end of this book you will know about a set
of skills and powers that enable any individual
to accomplish extraordinary things.

You will be able to use these skills and powers –
if you wish.

Much of the understanding that allows this is a distillation
of centuries of tradition and training, while other aspects
come from modern scientific or qualitative research.

Even after much editing, there is far too much of this
material to be accommodated in a book of this nature.

It is fascinating material, though. Consequently, we have
decided to dedicate a large part of the Calm Centre
web site to this 'surplus' material. You will see
references to it throughout the book.

You do not need this material to be able to use
Calm for Life **to its full potential.** The additional material
is provided for your interest or further study.

Please feel free to view this through the relevant web
address mentioned in the pages ahead. You will need
a password to gain access: that password is 'reader'.

Paul

INTRODUCTION

WHAT WILL IT TAKE?

Soon you're going to understand everything you will ever need to know about becoming calm for life.

You might wonder what sort of person could possibly know that.

Certainly not a scientist; they know too much about what is wrong with the world. And, through long associations with hospitals and research institutions, I know that many physicians and specialists are similarly burdened. That leaves academics, who usually have too much investment in the past, and political leaders, who often seem more governed by self-interest than vision.

Would an aspiring guru be more suited? After all, some of my most popular books have been about meditation – a topic much favoured by gurus. But gurus tend to focus on specific aspects of life, rather than all of life.

Would you heed a successful businessman? Or a television personality? Or a popular author?

I think not.

No, if there's any one reason why I should be the one to write a book called *Calm for Life,* it's because I know about calm.

Moreover, I know about it from endless perspectives. I've been researching this one topic for more than 20 years, and today employ several researchers working in this same area.

There is a wealth of information in this book. But, by the time you reach the end, your understanding about what it takes to be calm for life should amount to *more* than the sum of the information contained within these pages.

Let me show you how it works.

After many years of being involved with big business, I saw daily proof of the fact that information does not equate with knowledge. And, after just as many years of being involved with meditation, and to a lesser extent health, I realised that knowledge does not equal understanding.

The world is awash with data and information. The world's data bank doubles every few months or so. This flood of data is like the flood of radio signals that come to us from other galaxies: unrelenting, unending information which, in itself, does not mean a thing. Zilch. Just noise. Interference. Static. Blur.

But all is not wasted. Now and then a brilliant cosmologist comes along, analyses a few of these radio signals, and interprets what they mean. 'My God,' he splutters, 'these signals tell us that there is an object out there in the universe. It has zero volume, but infinite density!'

Now do you get it? This object has no mass at all. Even if you were right beside it, you wouldn't be able to see it, or hear it, or feel it. Yet it has infinite density.

Thankfully, someone like that cosmologist can take a garbled snippet of radio information and turn it into knowledge for us. He's described an object in space that has zero mass, but infinite density.

You mean you still don't get it?

Well, perhaps it's just a gap in your education. Perhaps if you were more scientifically inclined you might be able to derive understanding from that knowledge.

But you're still left scratching your head. 'Can't you see,' the cosmologist pleads, 'it's a black hole!'

But you still don't understand. And you know what? Nor does the overwhelming majority of the scientific community. They have the data; they have the knowledge; they have this beautiful metaphor; they suspect everyone else understands; but they themselves cannot comprehend anything described as a 'black hole'.

They're just like you and me.

Data is meaningless. Knowledge is only a part of the story. Understanding is everything.

Data is like bricks or building blocks. The bricks lie on the ground, get dusty, stop the grass from growing, but mean nothing much in their own right. Whether there are 1001 bricks or 1001^{10} bricks is irrelevant and, for the most part, meaningless. And it is not until someone comes along and puts them in order that you realise what you've been looking at is the makings of a brick wall.

Knowledge: Bricks = Wall.

Many people would be content with that knowledge. They can see a wall; their curiosity is satisfied. Now they know the meaning of bricks. But a more questioning person might very well ask, 'Why am I standing in front of a vast brick wall?'

Chances are, they will never understand this until they can see it from another perspective. Perhaps they could go into the stratosphere, look back and recognise it as the Great Wall of China – the world's largest construction, the only man-made structure visible from the moon. So they would have an understanding. Of sorts.

Someone else, a member of a 200 BC nomadic tribe from China's northern steppes, sees this same wall as an impenetrable barrier that will prevent him from attacking a rival tribe beyond the wall. Same data, same knowledge, yet another understanding.

Mr Fu, the tourist operator who buses thousands of German tourists to the wall each year, sees dollar signs on every brick. Once again, same data, same knowledge, but a completely different understanding.

Why I am pointing these things out is to explain the way I've chosen to write this book. I have included some data – not a lot, just enough to satisfy your curiosity. As well, I'll provide as much knowledge as I have been able to extract from all the volumes of data that pass through our hands.

But the understanding will have to come from you.

This will involve being open to what lies beyond the data, beyond the knowledge. But that's half the fun of the adventure we're about to embark on.

So, what will it take for you to be calm for life?

A quiet sense of inner peace that you can call upon, even on the busiest and most stressful occasions? Calm; no matter how bleak things may appear at certain times, no matter what state of health, employment or romantic entanglement you may find yourself in?

Perhaps your relationships play the key role in how calm and happy you can be. If so, rich, fulfilling, long-lasting relationships may be the most desirable outcome for bringing calm to your life.

Many people believe having sound health towers above all other needs. Combine this with boundless energy and an ever-present sense of optimism and adventure, and you may begin to appreciate the important role health can play in helping you to become calm for life. So why not include the ability to overcome illness and extend your lifespan at the same time?

Others would argue that spiritual fulfilment is more important.

Then again, you may think wealth, success and other worldly accomplishments are an integral part of what it takes to generate this ongoing peaceful state.

Maybe it's something entirely different.

What is important is that you have the choice. You get to choose any, or all, of these outcomes as a result of reading this book.

You may not appreciate it at this moment, but the further you delve into these pages, the clearer it will become to you: you do have the choice. And the further you go, the more choices will reveal themselves.

Calm for Life is a book of choices: at any stage you can settle for what you have read and taken out, or you can continue the journey.

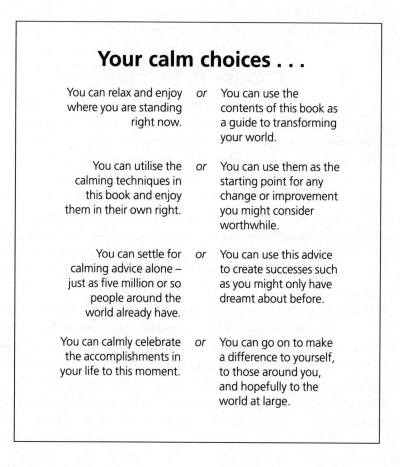

Your calm choices . . .

You can relax and enjoy where you are standing right now.	*or*	You can use the contents of this book as a guide to transforming your world.
You can utilise the calming techniques in this book and enjoy them in their own right.	*or*	You can use them as the starting point for any change or improvement you might consider worthwhile.
You can settle for calming advice alone – just as five million or so people around the world already have.	*or*	You can use this advice to create successes such as you might only have dreamt about before.
You can calmly celebrate the accomplishments in your life to this moment.	*or*	You can go on to make a difference to yourself, to those around you, and hopefully to the world at large.

Often, when faced with choices, you will wonder which is the right one, which is more appropriate. If you believe having too many choices can be just as stressful as having too few, relax: by the end of this book that pressure will not exist. You will discover there is no 'right' way to go, just as there is no wrong way. Either way can be made to work for you.

But, to remove any semblance of pressure, I've prepared a range of mechanisms that will have your decisions virtually making themselves for you. All you have to do is decide the overall direction that feels right, and there is even a simple technique for deciding that.

As for me, I've already made my choice. I've chosen to bring a little peace to your life. This will happen. And I do this in the hope that you might feel the urge to impart a little peace to somebody else, who in turn might pass it on . . .

Imagine what kind of life we could all have then.

Choose to be calm

Have you ever fantasised about being extremely rich, or extremely powerful? Be honest with yourself now. Have you ever fantasised about these possibilities? Just a little?

For most people, the underlying appeal of being rich or powerful is not the things they can possess or control, it is the choices such positions allow. If you're rich, you can choose to work or not, to be generous or not, to live wherever and however you feel. If you're powerful, you can choose to be magnanimous or demanding, to help others or not, to be respected or hated or feared. In other words, if you're rich or powerful, you believe you have more choices than if you're poor or weak.

Isn't it curious how you automatically begin to feel more relaxed and in control of your life, the moment you realise you have choices?

You see evidence of this every day of your life.

If someone says, 'You must do the morning shift,' you'll probably resent and possibly even resist this command. However, if they say, 'You can have the morning *or* the night shift,' you'll feel more comfortable about accepting the morning one. Why? Because you had the choice.

You see this in many contexts. In prisons, hospitals and nursing homes, for example, those who believe they have some choice in their menu – even though they receive essentially the same food as those who feel they have no choice – are significantly healthier, happier and more satisfied than those in the latter category.

When it comes to being calm, and feeling good about your work, your relationships and your life in general, you have choices. It may be difficult to accept this while you feel trapped in any particular work or lifestyle routine, but these choices exist.

It's not always easy to see this, but you have the power to be happy or unhappy, to be tense or relaxed, to be contented or depressed, to be rich or poor, to be well. Although doctors, psychologists, the media, schoolteachers and parents may try to convince you otherwise, you do have this power.

And, by the end of *Calm for Life*, this will be very, very clear to you.

1

THE AGE OF CALM

*You are about to discover
an extraordinary array of benefits
that arise when you can maintain
and utilise a unique sense
of inner calm . . .*

You live in an age where more data is gathered each hour than was gathered in the first few billion years of the world's existence. Today, the amount of information we file away each morning is exponentially greater than the amount we stored the day before. And the data snowball is just beginning to gather pace.

Yet, in spite of this immense accumulation of knowledge, we seem to know less than ever before.

Only 20 years ago we had a clear picture of who were the bad guys and who were the good guys in the world's armament race. Around 80 years before that everyone knew where good people went after they died; 100 years before that no-one ever asked why they had to work in a factory 7 days a week. And 800 years ago we knew what happened to sailors who ventured too far from our shores – they sailed over the edge. A few centuries before that we understood what caused floods, fires, locust plagues and meteorites – the gods were offended.

It seems like only yesterday that the answers dried up.

Our scientists, philosophers, politicians, gurus and spiritual leaders are every bit as certain as they have always been, yet our questions grow by the day.

'Why do I feel unsatisfied?'

'How can Rwandans be so brutal towards their neighbours?'

'Will I always feel this lonely?'

'When will someone work out a way of saving the ozone layer?'

In years gone by, people found their answers by looking to the past: ancient scriptures and teachings, traditional rituals and practices, superstitions.

In more recent times, the focus has shifted forwards – we have been convinced that science will discover solutions for all our health and ecological problems on some future occasion; we have been assured by a succession of political leaders and economists that economic growth will overcome all social ills; we have been seduced, cajoled, or motivated by self-help gurus (perhaps even myself included) into believing we can enjoy temporal and spiritual rewards we did nothing to deserve in the first place.

I suspect you already know that the answers you seek will come from someplace else. Soon you will either have these answers, or know exactly where to look to find them.

In the first instance, these answers will come from a few simple techniques that are not only easy to apply, but can be intensely pleasurable in their own right.

More importantly, many of these answers are ones that you already know. You may not be fully conscious of this yet, but some of them are within you now. Others will be answers you once had, but believed you had forgotten. One of the most charming letters I ever received from a reader made reference to this in relation to one of my earlier books: 'It contained so many of the things I had known and learned over the past forty years . . . but forgot last week'. Those words will have a special meaning to you by the end of this book.

Whether you have the answers now, or will know where to look for them soon, the fact is you are already well down the path to using them to get what you want out of life.

By the end of this book you will know what it takes to make the rest of your life calm, satisfying and filled with a sense of adventure. From a pleasantly relaxed state of mind, you will acquire new ways to improve your health, overcome illness, extend your years. If you are so inclined, you will even discover a calm, orderly approach to worldly gain – increasing wealth, achieving the 'impossible' and accomplishing virtually any objective you believe will make a difference.

These are big claims, I know. But there is a vast body of people who use these techniques – successfully, profitably and enjoyably – every day of their lives.

All made possible from a unique state of calm.

The spread of calm

Spreading calm is the purpose of my life's work.

For longer than I care to remember I have been researching, writing and lecturing on this topic. The early focus of my research was on calming techniques from India and, to a lesser extent, Taiwan, China, Tibet, Japan and Korea. My first book on this topic attempted to demystify many of the meditation styles and techniques from such countries for Western audiences. In the process my fascination for the centuries-old meditation practices grew to include the martial and healing arts as well.

This search brought me in contact with extraordinary people, some of whose teaching lineages dated back thousands of years.

Foremost among these was a master of Chi Kung ('Qigong' in Mandarin) I met in the mid-1970s when I first began investigating the martial arts. I still consider this man to be among the most inspiring people I have ever met.

My search had taken me to the Buddhist Po Lin monastery on the highest peak of Hong Kong's Lantau island. Even by my youthful standards the dormitory I was expected to sleep in was spartan. The beds were hard and wooden. Bright moonlight flooded in through the large, unclosing windows. As did droves of ferocious mosquitoes.

Finding sleep impossible, I sought sanctuary outside in the quiet, moonlit grounds. I was not alone. Around 3 a.m. is when the most devout exponents of Chi Kung and Wu Shu begin their exercises. On the cold paving before me was one such exponent: an extraordinary sight, he was graceful, powerful and amazingly supple. And, even though naked to the waist, he appeared impervious to the mosquitos.

He was short, bald and old – how old it was difficult to determine. One of his English-speaking colleagues assured me that he was born just after the second Opium War; this would have made him between 100 and 114 years old! Prior to his arrival in Hong Kong, he'd been an abbot in a monastery in the Yangtse Valley; fleeing China during the Cultural Revolution he'd taken refuge, unofficially, at Po Lin.

I made several efforts to trace him after that period, particularly after mainland China had reopened its doors to foreigners, but I never saw him again. This has in no way dulled my image of him. In spite of his years, my overriding memory is not of his age, nor his physical abilities; it is of the overwhelming sense of calm that emanated from him. You could not help but feel influenced by his serenity, and drawn into his state – where deadlines, responsibilities and worldly pressures simply did not exist.

Yet, at the same time, he positively bristled with energy. Here was a man you might expect to shuffle along, his aged joints creaking under the strain, yet he seemed to float about with his sandals barely touching the ground. Even though he was clearly an old man who spent much of his day in meditation, his body was as hard as the stone sleeping platform he lay on each night. And even though his eyesight was fading, he possessed the most subtle skills in acupuncture and herbalism. They said it was his training – after all, he was a master of Chi Kung, Tai Chi ('Taiji' in Mandarin) and just about every other healing and martial art I'd ever heard of. But I suspect it was more than that.

One of the skills he taught me shaped my life. It was not a martial art, nor was it any of the Tai Chi or Chi Kung techniques that could dictate the movement of chi within and without the body. It was a method of using the mind to effect changes in your self and the world around you.

He showed me how to use a specific state of inner calm to achieve things that extend way beyond most people's concept of 'achievable'. Whether this was a matter of strength, peace of mind, health, wealth or enlightenment, the boundaries could be endlessly extended.

This ability – to go to a place deep within yourself and harness *all* of your physical, emotional, psychological, intuitive and spiritual forces in order to accomplish something beyond the limits of perceived human capabilities – could be seen as a superhuman ability.

Yet, in reality, it is a very human ability. It can be taught. It can be learned. It can be applied.

You may have seen it applied when martial artists concentrate all their chi into one part of their body, so that it can withstand any physical force – a fist, a sword, a sledgehammer. Or when they deliver awesome force with a single blow.

You may have seen it applied when a yogi goes into a state of deep meditation – lowering their pulse and breathing rates to levels that alarm medically trained people – and suddenly becomes aware of events and understandings that are beyond our rational observation.

You may have heard about it being applied when individuals make unexplained recoveries from life-threatening or 'terminal' illnesses.

Or when physicists go beyond conventional understanding to discover earthly and universal matters that change forever the course of scientific practice.

Or when sportspeople overcome great setbacks to rewrite the rule books in athletic achievement.

Or when artists or musicians create moments so inspired and magical that you feel some sort of divine influence is at play.

Or when people learn how to be calm or happy – at will.

These are not miracles. They are not necessarily the actions of geniuses or those with superhuman powers. Nor are they freak, unre-producible occurrences. They are simple, practical, achievable products of a unique state of calm – one that everyday human beings like you and me can enter.

Everyone?

Traditionally, there have been two impediments to achieving this: very few people, either Eastern or Western, knew about it; it required many years of dedicated practice.

It has long been believed that the only people capable of attaining the state of inner calm I write of are experienced meditators – by which I mean those who have been practising it for more than 20 years. People such as this can attain a unique physiological state (referred to as the yogic state) after 5–10 minutes of concentration. Naturally, not everyone is prepared to invest those 20 years or so in order to create the kind of life they want for themselves, no matter how fantastic that potential life may be.

I might still have been discussing this on the theoretical level but for a breakthrough, 4 or 5 years ago, when one of my researchers pointed out that a technique I had been teaching could short-circuit the process, turning it into a half-hour exercise. Unknowingly, I had been using it all along. It not only enabled me to effect a profoundly calm state – more or less at will – but also could be easily taught to others.

By the end of this book, you will have this skill.

Half an hour for life

Have you ever considered that high-achievers in business might have something in common with world-champion boxers? And that best-selling authors might employ similar 'accomplishment strategies' to people who cure themselves of life-threatening illnesses? Is it possible that Formula 1 drivers and great opera singers draw on similar internal resources when they reach the peak of their performance? What about chefs, martial artists, derivatives traders, religious leaders, entrepreneurs, politicians and jockeys?

Not only is this similarity possible, it's almost surely so.

In recent years I've met many highly accomplished people, the overwhelming majority of whom use a surprisingly similar 'accomplishment strategy': first, effect a state of inner calm, then use that state to achieve what you want to achieve.

Why aren't you aware of this? Probably because they aren't aware of it themselves.

But now that it has been pointed out, observe any major achiever in the moments before they hit the high point, and you will see a small pause . . . where they become still. If you're close enough, you'll notice their eyes get a distant look in them. And, even though their pulse may be racing with anticipation, they will be experiencing a sense of deep inner calm.

That is the first step.

If you get nothing more from *Calm for Life* than learning how to master this first step, it will have served you well. And you will be well on the way to bringing peace, harmony and contentment to your life.

If you want more, there are techniques in this book that use a state of inner calm to enable you to accomplish whatever you believe is important. These have been derived from my research into the various self-transforming arts of the East and West; studies of outstanding successes in the fields of business, healing, learning, arts and sport; and years of involvement at the highest levels of corporate, government, medical and business worlds.

Yet it is not essential to pursue or to realise what some believe are the 'big' achievements. So often these have more to do with others' goals and expectations than they do with our own. And trying to conform or measure up to others' standards is a sure recipe for failure. (Some psychologists believe *all* thoughts that lead to depression stem from our tendency to compare ourselves and our circumstances with others; if we compare well, we feel uplifted, but if we compare poorly, we feel depressed.)

This book will show you how to filter those expectations so they are specific to you and your needs.

You may decide that the greatest achievement in life is simply being calm, happy and fulfilled. I know many 'successful' people who would give everything they have for these basic qualities of life.

Soon you will know how to attain them. Easily.

The benefits of calm

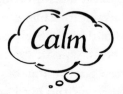

Calm. Notice how the mere appearance of that word is enough to start you feeling relaxed? Try saying it to yourself. 'Calm.' Notice how the sound of the word immediately begins to ease you into a calmer state? Notice how the thought has begun to relax you – already?

Calm is an extraordinarily powerful word in its own right. Without even delving into its meaning, it has an immediate and quite noticeable calming effect on people.

For me, this effect is never more pronounced than when I'm doing television or radio interviews. Time after time I'll walk into the studio, find everyone in a rush getting the program together, ushering guests in and out; the interviewer will be distracted and tense, sipping coffee, adjusting their wardrobe, and trying to keep abreast of all the things that are going on at the same time. One glance at this environment, one glance at the producer and the interviewer, and you'd be convinced that nothing on earth could ever induce them to unwind.

Then, a transformation takes place. Within seconds of starting the conversation about calm, an unmistakeable change of pace occurs. The interviewer's gestures become more relaxed. If you pay attention, you'll notice how their breathing rate slows down. Quite slow, deep, relaxed. And the pace of their words begins to slow down as well. And, before you know it, a tense, high-energy interviewer is transformed into a model of calm. You can probably imagine how powerfully this begins to work: slow words, slow gestures, slow breathing . . .

You see, just the discussion of calm helps people to become calm. Often, no other effort is required. Just the discussion.

Many years ago, I conducted a study into the physiological impact of words used as mantras for meditation. Conventional wisdom in those days (and it's still widely promoted today) is that certain words or expressions – usually chosen from the Vedas (Hindu scriptures) or other religious writings – were more potent than words from our everyday language.

In this study, a range of phrases was given to various meditators and *subjective* evaluations of the effectiveness of these words were sought after intervals of 90 days, 12 months, 24 months and 36 months. The words included: 'smith', 'tan', 'singh' (words from the phone book), 'Om' and a range of popular Sanskrit phrases used as mantras in the Tantric malas (rosaries); and 'calm'. Also included were a number of personal mantras that had been given to individual students by their meditation teachers.

Except for those using personal mantras, who had already made a degree of commitment to these, the simple word 'calm' came out on top – that is, users found this the most calming and *pleasing* word for both short- and long-term use in meditation. (I make no claims for its spiritual effectiveness.)

So much for words. But what about calm itself? Do we actually need calm? Is it good for us? Does it enrich our lives?

Before I go on to the benefits of knowing how to become calm, we might consider what it means to be calm. The calm that I advocate is not necessarily a lazy, inactive state of lethargy or rest: it's a state of mind, a state of *inner* calm. The same state that great athletes employ at the beginning of an event; the same state that martial artists strive to attain during even the most aggressive contests; the same state that actors, boxers, musicians, surgeons, businesspeople and psychologists strive to maintain while they go about their business.

This is what being calm is about. It is about being able to enjoy a peaceful sense of order and control while you go about the normal events of your busy, demanding life . . . so that you can get more satisfaction out of your busy, demanding life . . . so that you can achieve more in your busy, demanding life. And, over and above all that, so that you can *enjoy* your busy, demanding life.

Knowing how to become calm – at will – will help you restore your sense of wellbeing when things go wrong. It will help you cope with the stresses and pressures you face each day. And it will help you to appreciate that life is a wondrous experience, even as those around you fret about the world economy, the population explosion, meteor showers, rogue hedge funds, the depletion of the ozone layer, pirates in the South China Sea and the price of organic vegetables.

This seemingly idyllic state is achievable when you know how to cultivate and maintain a state of inner calm at all times.

By the end of this book, you will know this.

Calm for its own sake

Foremost among the benefits that flow from being calm is one that the stress-management industry continually overlooks. That is, that being calm can be a pleasure in its own right.

We live in an over-stimulated society, where advertising and consumerism have convinced us that the only worthwhile state in life is stimulation. Advertisers, marketers and the media have trained us to believe that if we're not being stimulated, we're missing out on something.

There was a time – not so very long ago – when our lives fluctuated between two different states, stimulation and relaxation. Most people sought a balance between the two: some of the time stimulated, some of the time relaxed. These days, the emphasis in life is on stimulation. Indeed, we have now reached the farcical stage where many people seek stimulation . . . for their relaxation! They do this in the mistaken belief that more and more novel forms of stimulating activities constitute, by some odd twist of logic, a form of relaxation.

Clearly, we have a contradiction in terms here. Stimulation is the opposite of relaxation. Only relaxation is relaxation. Stimulation is designed to excite and titillate the senses and nervous system; relaxation is designed to calm them.

Do you see the paradox?

We've been so conditioned to seek greater and greater levels of stimulation in our everyday lives – from the moment we turn on the radio in the morning, to the Walkman on your run, to the slogans on your public transport, to the animated screensavers on your computer, to the spicy food at lunch, to the magazine on the bus coming home, to the television program at night, to the CD as we're preparing for bed – that we've forgotten there is another aspect to being human. Instead of human beings, we've become human *doings*. This conditioning has been so thorough that we've reached the stage where a significant pro-portion of the developed world's population now views an absence of stimulation as a negative state.

Is it any wonder we're restless? What a belief to instil in our children!

So, let's slow down for a moment and consider the pleasure and desirability of relaxation. Of being relaxed.

The pleasure of calm

Here's something you can do tonight to prove to yourself how pleasurable the simple act of being calm can be.

- Run a warm bath.
- Throw in those expensive bath salts you've been saving for a special occasion – or add five drops of lavender and rose oils.
- Light a candle, turn off the lights.
- Take a warm face towel and drape it over your face as you sink down into the tub.
- Tell yourself you have all the time in the world. Then listen to the sound of your relaxed breath-ing as you begin to forget there's another world outside.

How many times in your life have you looked back on a leisurely, non-stimulating experience of some kind and thought, 'I really enjoyed that'? How often have you gone for a walk along a deserted beach or through a quiet park by yourself – not actively 'having fun', not encountering anything unexpected, nor learning anything of particular importance – then looked back on the experience as one of the more pleasant and enriching activities of your week? How often have you walked away from a party or a television program to sit under a tree in the garden, then wondered why you don't do this sort of thing more often?

Once you recall these events, you'll appreciate that being calm or relaxed is a pleasure in its own right. It is not an entertainment, it is not a form of stimulation, it is not something that you plan with nervous anticipation. But it is a pleasure.

So I'm asking you to keep this thought in your mind for the duration of this book: *being calm is a pleasure in its own right.*

It is not a chore, an obligation, or a regime you have to adhere to. It is simply a pleasure. Sheer, unadulterated, guilt-free pleasure. Indeed, to be absolutely relaxed and peaceful is one of the most rewarding, most uplifting experiences a human being can have.

You've probably already begun to realise – if not consciously, then somewhere within your subconscious – that being calm is one of the simplest, and surest, ways to feel good. And that while you're feeling good, it's impossible to feel stressed or on edge. Can you imagine how relaxed you'd be feeling now if you'd known that all along?

Calm for adjustment or remedy

In spite of the pleasure and the cosy feeling that came over you when you first thought of this topic, calm will usually be considered in the same context as stress. While I could quite happily go through life without drawing any further attention to this subject, it will probably arise in your thoughts, so I'd better address it.

Yes, we live in a stressful age. Is it more stressful than when the average life expectancy was 49 years, children worked down the mines, and adults worked 7 days a week in uncomfortable, sometimes dangerous conditions? I believe so.

To many of us, today's world is a pretty scary place. Insecurity rules. So many of the standards and practices that we used to know and take for granted are fast becoming history. Social values are changing; so too are the workplace, family structure, our population mix, and our attitudes to health, relationships and morality. And one of the few certainties in life is that things are going to change even more. Change is one of today's most prevalent stressors.

Even our worries are changing. Instead of worrying about who they're going to play with after school, children worry about the state of the planet; teachers worry about trends in the world economy; and school principals are more concerned about syringes than they are about science.

Let's stop talking in abstract terms for a moment. What about you? Is your life improving the way you want it to? Are you growing more peaceful and fulfilled by the day, or are you feeling progressively more anxious about what lies ahead? Are you concerned about job security? Maybe you don't have a job at all, or you are working too hard and feel guilty about not spending enough quality time with your children.

Another unsettling influence today is the omnipresence of the media. We cannot get through a day without being harangued by what's going wrong in the world – in newspaper headlines, television newsflashes, electronic billboards, radio news bulletins, phone messages while you're on hold, and even via our computer monitors. Where once our concerns would have been limited to the goings on in our neighbourhood or town, we now have concerns about things going on in places that, in another age, we might never even have known existed. Is it any wonder you feel unsettled knowing that 1200 miners are trapped underground in Angola, that a woman on the space shuttle is suffering from peritonitis and requires an immediate appendectomy, that 2 million land mines are buried in Afghanistan, that the crops have failed in Honduras, that there's widespread flooding in India, that the polar ice cap is melting, and that people in Western nations are getting fatter by the day? It is natural for us to be concerned about these calamities; and it makes us even more concerned when we realise there is absolutely nothing we can do to overcome them.

But you *can* control the way they affect you.

A few days ago I read a magazine with the words 'The Stress Epidemic' emblazoned across its cover. It was in red type; it's always in red type. It seems as if every few months a magazine or daily news-paper opens up the files and says, 'We haven't used this one for a while', and drags out the same tired old line. Not only is this unimaginative and alarmist, it succeeds in creating a worse problem than the one it's attempting to draw its readers' attention to. Besides, it's a dreadful cliché.

Recently, at a conference in Hawaii, I met a public relations executive who claimed to have written the original version of that line – in a press release for a well-known antidepressant. If this is true, we can see the vested interest at work here. My strong belief is that the discussion of stress, and especially its associated symptoms, only serves to add to the stresses of life.

Please remember that it is perfectly natural for you to experience the stresses of modern life. Perfectly natural. These stresses do exist and, just as surely, will continue to exist. It is the height of folly to think you can eliminate them. But, by learning how to become calm – and to use this state whenever you need to – you can eliminate, or lessen, the impact these stresses have on you. You can find simple, enjoyable ways of dealing with life's ups and downs without necessarily succumbing to illness, unhappiness, Prozac, breakdown, divorce or therapy.

You may not be aware of it yet, but you are already a considerable way along the path towards achieving this. A powerful, pleasurable state of inner calm is now well within your reach.

The technical view of stress

Technically speaking, there are three different types of stresses in life: mechanical stresses, chemical stresses and emotional stresses. In the context of a book like this, you would probably lump these into two areas: physical stresses (mechanical and chemical) and emotional stresses.

Mechanical stress   The deformation of a physical object produces both stress and strain. The applied stress (or the load) is directly proportional to the strain. When the applied stress reaches a stage where the strain is no longer reversible (the yield point), the result is permanent strain or fracture.

You can easily relate to this. If someone twists your arm behind your back (a stress), you will feel the strain; but you are relieved to discover that your arm returns to normal the moment the stress is removed. However, if someone twists your arm all the way to the yield point, you end up with a permanent strain or fracture – a ruptured tendon or broken arm.

Chemical stress   Although we may not be fully aware of them, chemical stresses can be a major strain on our health and wellbeing.

Such stresses arise from chemicals in the atmosphere (air pollution); chemicals in the food chain (additives, pesticides); chemicals in our day-to-day environment (from air-conditioning, photocopiers, household chemicals, insecticides); chemicals we willingly imbibe (nicotine, caffeine, alcohol); and ones I call 'personal chemicals' (deodorants, synthetic clothing, make-up and so on).

The use of such chemicals has become so pronounced that today it is estimated that every living organism on this planet contains about 500 chemicals that are not part of its natural system. At least some of these uninvited chemicals must be considered stressors.

Emotional stress This is the one you know best of all. Emotional stress is the area the magazines write their 'stress epidemic' articles about. These are the stresses that are a product of what's inside your head rather than what's happening in the world around you – though usually it will appear otherwise.

Emotional stressors are the most difficult to deal with, since they are often subtle or go unnoticed until such time as they create problems for you. For this reason, they are usually the most pervasive and most damaging, especially over the longer term.

My view of stress

Accepting that there are physical and emotional stresses, we can now concentrate on the stresses that relate to you, your attitudes and the way you approach life.

In my earlier books, I divided the major stressors into categories that related to specific areas of life – such as the workplace in *Calm at Work*. This book takes a much broader perspective on life. So, taking this broader perspective, I believe all emotional stresses of modern life fall into three categories. These relate to time, space and order.

Appropriately, all are overcome by using the same approach.

Time Go up to anyone in the street and ask what the main cause of pressure in their life is, and chances are they'll say 'time'. As the world gets busier, as the demands from your work and acquaintances rise, it becomes increasingly obvious that the one thing in life you have no control over is time.

This should not be difficult to understand. From the very earliest age we are being programmed to be time-conscious – 'Hurry up, Paul, or you'll miss the bus', 'Get a move on, we're running late', 'Why are you always late?' Punctuality rates with honesty as a mark of character. So we go through life believing there is more and more we have to accomplish in the time we have available – that is, the time we have available in our working day and the time we have left on this planet (or so we believe).

But that's only one aspect of time pressure. Another aspect relates to time that has passed. Regrets about things you should have said or done, but didn't. Guilt over transgressions that should have been long forgotten. Sadness over events that happened long ago. Anger about matters that have never been resolved. Disappointment over relationships that go back to your childhood. Limiting beliefs learnt at the earliest age.

All of these relate to the past – an aspect of time that, at this very moment, has no relevance whatsoever. (If you've suffered badly over past wrongs, you may baulk at this suggestion, claiming you are a product of your past. But *at this very moment*, the past does not exist.)

Another aspect of time relates to things that are not happening, have never happened, and probably never will. This is known as anxiety. Worry and anxiety are always future-based. They relate to events or outcomes which, on average, never even come close to eventuating. Most worries, most anxieties, are fictions.

There is just one moment in time when you can have no regrets about the past, nor any concerns about the future. That moment is 'NOW'. Even if the past and future are a continuum, the point where they meet is NOW.

NOW is not something you can think about or analyse while you are experiencing it. It just happens. Right now, time has no beginning or end, and exerts no pressure. This is why the experience of NOW precludes stressful thoughts. NOW is the easiest state to attain, yet is one of the most desirable states imaginable.

Space   Space relates to our physical world, where we encounter a range of stresses, such as noise pollution.

Space plays a powerful psychological role in our lives. You can see this in cities. Broadly speaking, large cities fall into two categories: vertical cities such as New York and Hong Kong, and horizontal cities such as Los Angeles and Sydney. The vertical cities cram increasing numbers of people onto the same small 'footprint' and tend to be more tense in atmosphere; their residents report high personal stress levels, and interpersonal behaviour appears to be more aggressive. Horizontal cities, on the other hand, have more of a feeling of space about them as they distribute their populations outwards. The subjective experience of residents of such cities is slightly more relaxed than those of their counterparts in vertical cities. Of course, both types of cities have horizontal as well as vertical attributes, but one or other usually dominates.

Is this difference in tension levels real or perceived? Evidence suggests that it is a perception. If you compare the 'tension statistics' of both types of cities – the rates of violent crime, suicides, mental disorders, alcoholism and drug addiction – rates do not reflect the density so much as the sheer numbers of the population. Nevertheless, the individual's perception is that vertical cities increase the pressure and strain of everyday life. This is understandable: stress levels escalate when you are forced to share limited personal space. When you house too many rats in a cage, they become frustrated, aggressive, and their lifespan is shortened. You also see frustration and aggression when you squeeze too many people into a confined office space, or force too many commuters onto a train, or cram students into a classroom.

Conversely, if you could be transported to a wide open field or a deserted beach right now, you would feel calmer, less aggressive and more at peace (assuming you are not agoraphobic). Space creates calm. Congestion creates tension.

Similarly, where you are located in relation to the events going on in your life influences the way you feel. If you believe you are standing at the point of intersection of hundreds of life's dramas, you will feel trapped and tense; whereas if you believe you are standing way off in the distance watching them go by, you will be calmer. Space in this sense is metaphoric rather than actual, but it still creates the same effect.

Knowing this enables you to utilise certain mental techniques that can help you relax, no matter how congested your environment. Paradoxically, the more centred you feel when you're in these environments of limited space, the calmer you feel. We will explore this in more detail later.

Order   Most of us struggle to maintain a sense of order in our world. We cling to the things we have. We try to control the attitudes and actions of those around us so that they align with our own. We resent those who are different from us, those who challenge our standards or the status quo.

In striving to preserve this order – or this perception of order – we create stresses for ourselves. Why? Because, as far as we know, order cannot be preserved; it gives way to chaos in an almost predictable fashion. In addition to this, the world most of us live in is linear: a world of measurements and straight lines. We take comfort from things that conform and add up. We believe all questions must have answers. This linearity extends to the events of our lives. Since childhood, we've been taught that all good stories have a beginning, a middle and an end; that crime does not pay, all good is rewarded, and chosen people live happily ever after.

Not surprisingly, our expectation of the world is very close to that. And when the events of our lives do not progress in this orderly, understandable fashion, we become frustrated. Stressed.

The belief that we have no control over the important areas of our lives – work, relationships, health, fortunes – is possibly the most damaging source of emotional stress in our lives. The struggle to maintain order in a universe that is inherently chaotic only emphasises that lack of control. It is not easy to accept change, especially when you are content with what you have, but change is the order of the day.

Accepting the chaos is the key to becoming calm. And the calmest place amidst the chaos is right in the centre.

Look at yourself

It may help at this stage if we pause to take a look at the way your body and your emotions react to stressful situations. There was a time when people spoke of their vulnerability to life's stresses as 'having nerves', or even 'suffering from nerves'. As quaint as this expression may be, it has a strong biological foundation.

Your peripheral nervous system has two distinct sub-systems: the somatic system, which regulates your external or voluntary actions; and the autonomic system, which is concerned with your internal organs and involuntary actions. The autonomic system is further divided into the sympathetic and parasympathetic nervous systems.

The sympathetic nervous system is active all of the time and helps you meet the demands of a busy, active life. It is designed to prepare you for emergency action ('fight or flight') – speeding up your heart rate and blood flow, tensing your muscles, increasing perspiration, pumping adrenal hormones such as adrenalin and corticosteroids into the system. Stimulation of this sympathetic nervous system is usually accompanied by feelings of tension or fear, such as a sick or sinking feeling in the stomach.

Now we come to its counterpart, the parasympathetic nervous system. Under ideal circumstances, this comes into play after your sympathetic system has played its part. The parasympathetic system is the restorer, the balancer, the healer, the energy conserver. It's the one designed to calm you down after those moments of arousal or action, and to return you to your normal state. Overall, its function is recovery – to prepare you for another burst of 'emergency' action.

If you compare the attributes of the sympathetic nervous response with the well-known 'symptoms of stress', you'll see a surprising correlation between the two. These symptoms include:

- Breathing difficulties
- Butterflies in the stomach
- Clenched fingers
- Cold, clammy hands
- Dry mouth
- Feeling faint
- Fidgeting
- Indigestion
- Loss of appetite
- Palpitations
- Rapid pulse
- Speeded-up conversation
- Stiff neck or shoulders
- Tightness in the stomach or chest wall
- Trembling hands

Clearly, all those alarming characteristics the stress therapists caution you about may not be so alarming after all – they're perfectly normal characteristics of a functioning sympathetic nervous system.

One of the peculiarities of the sympathetic nervous system is the wholehearted way it functions. When it's operating, it's really operating! 100 percent. All organs playing. This is perfectly normal. *It only departs from the norm when there is no relief at the conclusion of these efforts.*

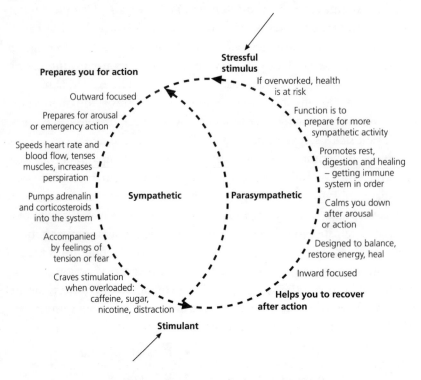

Prepares you for action

Stressful stimulus

If overworked, health is at risk

Outward focused

Function is to prepare for more sympathetic activity

Prepares for arousal or emergency action

Speeds heart rate and blood flow, tenses muscles, increases perspiration

Promotes rest, digestion and healing – getting immune system in order

Sympathetic   **Parasympathetic**

Pumps adrenalin and corticosteroids into the system

Calms you down after arousal or action

Accompanied by feelings of tension or fear

Designed to balance, restore energy, heal

Inward focused

Craves stimulation when overloaded: caffeine, sugar, nicotine, distraction

Helps you to recover after action

Stimulant

Sympathetic and parasympathetic nervous systems

You can see from the diagram above that if you overwork your sympathetic nervous system – that is, subject yourself to continuous stresses without adequate recuperation in between – it tends to become self-energising. First of all it creates a craving for stimulants: you reach for a coffee, a Mars bar, or a cigarette, then these stimulants re-energise the sympathetic nervous system and provide the fuel to start the whole stressful cycle again.

This is where stress problems begin to develop. The adrenal glands continue to pump adrenalin and corticosteroids into your body in an effort to help your body adapt to the stress. Eventually this process *appears* to calm you down, but it is an illusion; your system does not return to normal. Moreover, this response also serves to inhibit the effectiveness of your immune system, leaving you vulnerable to disease and illness. And that's only part of the story. If your parasympathetic system fails to calm you down, cortisol continues to be pumped into your system until it reaches the stage where it can cause damage to the parts of your brain that control your emotions, learning and memory. You might be able to imagine where *that* leads . . .

Because practices such as yoga and meditation replicate the actions of your parasympathetic nervous system, you can see how they might improve the efficiency of your immune system. And why they help fight and overcome illness.

(Incidentally, I have encountered a few headline-seekers in various countries pushing a 'stress is good for you' agenda in recent times. These people seem to be motivated by the shock value of their theses. There is, in fact, a wealth of information showing that undergoing extended episodes of stress, or indeed any stimulation of the nervous system, has a negative effect on the immune system – in some cases causing permanent harm.)

However, while it is true that today's world can be stressful and that many of its stresses are unavoidable, we should not be fooled into thinking there is such a medical or psychological condition as 'stress'. While there are often specific reactions that follow stressful events, such as post-traumatic stress and post-operative stress, I do not accept that stress is a psychological condition comparable with schizophrenia or manic depression, or a physical condition like herpes, tonsillitis or dandruff.

The problem is not stress but the way we react to stressful events, the way we think and the habits we develop. If we exclude the real traumas – deaths, divorces, assault, arrest and so on – we find that most of the stresses we face are relatively mundane, and often similar.

We all have 24 hours in our day. We all have bosses, partners, shareholders or publishers who expect too much from us during those hours. We all have to contend with noisy children and reckless drivers from time to time. The difference between one person and another in these circumstances is the way they react. One person shakes their head at the reckless driver, then smiles, thinking how fortunate they are not to be in such a rush; another person curses under their breath, and spends the rest of the day thinking about how they'd like to get even. The same stressor (a reckless driver) in both cases, but two totally different reactions.

Stress itself is not the condition; it is the inability to cope with stress that causes other conditions to develop. This inability to cope leads to three stages of deterioration:

Stage	Effects	Feeling	Treatment
1	A succession of stressful incidents, conditions or behaviour	This is what most people would refer to as 'feeling stressed'.	This can be remedied by an awareness of what's going on, combined with a range of pleasurable calming techniques.
2	Generalised feelings of anxiety	By this stage, a person feels a sense of disquiet about the future, but cannot think of any logical reason why this should be so.	A more thorough effort is required here – such as a commitment to exercise and meditation programs, combined with a change in the way life's stresses are viewed.
3	Loss of emotional control	This is the most difficult stage – where a person feels they cannot cope with the event, or the world at large, any longer.	This requires an ongoing commitment to several calming programs (such as those in Chapter 6), and perhaps professional assistance.

If you are suffering from these effects of stress, it's not your fault. The media is continually telling us what's wrong with the world, producing mental stress; the weather patterns are more erratic than any of us can recall (physical stress); and, considering the number of uninvited chemicals that find their way into your body, you're prob-ably being poisoned as well (chemical stress).

Of course, not all stress is deleterious to your health. To simplify: stress can be either negative or positive.

By my definition, negative stresses are those that you have little or no control over. These include physical stresses such as noisy work environments or strained eyesight; mental stresses such as loneliness or financial worries; and chemical stresses such as poor diet or air pollution. Unresolved over the longer term, they tend to have a neg-ative effect on your mood and your health.

Positive stresses, on the other hand, are exciting. These are the activities you often initiate for yourself – the football game, the roller coaster ride, the early days of a love affair. Even laughter.

While the sympathetic nervous system initially responds to these positive stresses in the same way as it does to negative stresses, the after-effects are different. They *enhance* your immune system and restore your sense of wellbeing. In other words, they are life-enriching.

Take laughter, for example. When you laugh, your endocrine sys-tem releases substances which relax you, suppress pain, help stabilise your blood pressure, and aid your digestion and circulation. Laughter is a positive stress. Have a laugh, enjoy yourself – and not only will you feel like living longer, but you probably will live longer.

The healing power of calm

We know that too much exposure to psychological stress makes a person more susceptible to physical illness – from colds through to more serious conditions such as heart disease, stroke and even cancer. We also know that stress has been directly linked to conditions such as hypertension. And that wounds take longer to heal when a person is subjected to stressful conditions.

Now we are beginning to discover that the opposite state to stress – calm – plays a powerful role in countering these effects. A calm state helps to maintain wellness, speeds recovery from illness and gen-erally assists in all aspects of healing. It is no coincidence that so many progressive cancer clinics now include meditation, or meditation-type techniques, as part of their therapy. Why? Because they have seen that patients who utilise these techniques have significantly better survival rates, and better recovery rates, than those who don't.

Please bear in mind that I am being deliberately moderate in these claims. There are hundreds of successful doctors and therapists who make much greater claims for the healing power of meditation and relaxation therapies than those you've just read. I know many individuals who have used specific calming techniques to overcome so-called incurable illnesses: 22 years ago, one of my close friends used the calming methods of Chi Kung to overcome 'terminal' throat cancer. He is still fit and well today.

But does being calm cure illness?

Not directly. But being calm does help the immune system, and a fully functioning immune system is a formidable ally in the healing process. This is neither speculation nor the wishful thinking of some alternative practitioners. A wealth of research has been conducted into the link between mental and emotional states and the immune system – and we now know that at stressful times, the brain and all organs involved in the immune system act as an integrated whole.

So science can now clearly show that your thoughts and attitudes play a major role in your health. (You've probably known this all along.)

Calm for balance

We know that calm is enjoyable in its own right. We know that it strengthens your body's immunity against disease. We also know that it can assist in the healing process. But probably its most appealing benefit is the way it helps you to get more out of life.

When you know how to maintain a sense of inner calm, you will be:

- better able to cope with everyday problems

- emotionally more resilient

- happier and more optimistic

- more energetic and mentally alert

- more creative

- more tolerant.

And you'll probably sleep better, eat better, and be more enthusiastic about life.

In the past, most of the evidence for this was anecdotal. However,
not so long ago, one of the Calm Centre's researchers conducted a
survey into attitudes in the workplace, to see if there was any significant connection between different emotional states and
performance. (See page 98 for some background on the Calm Centre
and its aims.)

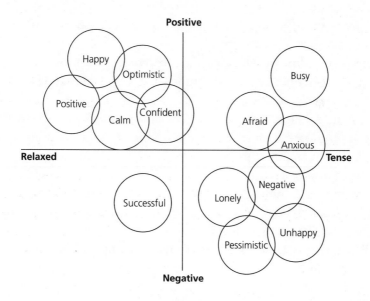

Emotion 'clusters' in the workplace

One aspect of this study that we found revealing was the 'clusters'
of emotions that occurred. For example, 'calm' people tended to share
happy, optimistic and confident characteristics; while 'anxious' people
were more inclined to feel unhappy and negative. ('Successful' and
'busy' tended to occupy territories of their own.) In addition, most
people who described themselves as being calm also described themselves as being positive.

By the end of this book, you will not only be feeling calmer, but
much more positive. And you will be awash with new ways of using
calm to exert a positive influence on your own health and mental
wellbeing.

Calm for change

Now we come to the benefit that I've been hesitating to write about for almost 20 years.

It's about how you can use a specific state of inner calm to transform yourself, or to achieve whatever you believe is worthwhile. And whether your ambition is a physical one, an emotional one, or one of accomplishment in any particular field, you can throw away the rule book. The possibilities are virtually unlimited.

I am not exaggerating. I have seen this capability demonstrated literally hundreds of times in recent years.

Some will find it difficult to accept what I am proposing. Then again, some people believe it is impossible for a bare-handed man to break several housebricks with his palm; for a person over-loaded with responsibilities to feel they have all the time in the world; for a person diagnosed with terminal illness to recover; or for an impoverished, poorly educated person to become a world leader.

But consider this: not so very long ago, many believed it was impossible for a human being to run a mile in under 4 minutes, or to set foot on the moon, or to sail too far north without dropping off the edge of the earth.

What this suggests is that one person's impossibility is another person's challenge.

And it does not take superhuman strength, education, position, intellect or privilege; all it takes are a few simple techniques, and the launching point of a state of inner calm.

While I am excited by the possibilities I'm going to tell you about, they are almost commonplace to me now. In my own circle of acquaintances are people who have used these techniques to achieve what conventional wisdom said was unachievable:

- A 65-year-old man in need of income who entered a new field, and made millions out of an idea designed to educate children about conservation.

- A writer who, after decades of lunch-money-sized book advances, suddenly moved into the million-per-book league. (Not me, unfortunately!)

- A woman who, inspired by the desire to serve, rose from obscurity to lead one of the world's few matriarchal religions.

- A man who wasn't a professional writer but became one of the world's biggest-selling authors for 2 years in a row.

- A martial artist who abandoned 1000 years of tradition, and now leading exponents of *all* martial arts make the pilgrimage to his academy to study his art.

- A young Russian athlete who became a feared opponent and a world boxing champion without ever getting angry.

- A young Texan who became the first non-Japanese recognised as a Grand Master in the shakuhachi (Zen flute) tradition.

- Innumerable determined individuals who have overcome life-threatening and so-called 'terminal' illnesses.

(More details of some of these transformations are available on the Calm Centre's web site at www.calmcentre.com/reader; you'll need the password 'reader'.)

Most people who know these individuals would have said these achievements were either impossible or highly improbable. And would have warned against pursuing them.

Yet, those who are familiar with the state of inner calm about which I write will find it easy to accept. Without exception, these people approached their success from a very similar state – a deeply relaxed state that I call Deep Calm, plus one other attribute that I will explain to you later in this book.

You might quite justifiably think: 'Maybe these were exceptional people in the first place. It is easy for exceptional people to accomplish out-of-the-ordinary things.' Considering that most of these people were from my own circle of acquaintances (at least initially), I can vouch for the fact many of them were of modest abilities or education.

Reading that, you'll probably wonder whether Paul Wilson's concept of 'modest' coincides with your own. I wondered this myself – did I naturally gravitate towards people who were going to achieve momentous things for themselves, or for others?

So I started to examine the lives of others I believed to be successful, whose accomplishments rose above the everyday. These were not just material successes I was interested in, but accomplishments in all aspects of life – relationships, living, thinking, caring. When I could finally afford my own researchers, we interviewed people who'd enjoyed beautiful relationships for 50 years, and still gave thanks for every moment they were allowed to spend with their partners. We interviewed people who'd quietly devoted their lives to helping others – medically, materially and spiritually. We interviewed people whose thoughts and perspectives on life were an inspiration to those around them. And, naturally, we interviewed those who'd reached the top in sport, arts, business and public service.

Almost all these people had something in common. And, even today, I never cease to be amazed at just how easy it seemed for them to accomplish what they did. This is not to suggest they had an easy time of it. Examine their life stories and you might blanch at the pain, the setbacks and the bankruptcies they had to endure on the way. Just as all people do. But the *accomplishments* of their lives were – relatively speaking – easy.

Why? Because they made the decision not to be bound by the normal constraints that most of us believe we are constrained by.

At the risk of being repetitive, I would like to emphasise this point: we are constrained by what we *believe* we are constrained by.

The moment you realise this, you are faced with unlimited potential.

So far you've discovered that:

- **Calm can be scientifically shown to enhance healing and the immune system.**
- **Being calm is a choice.**
- **It is easy to become calm – at will.**
- **From this calm state you can achieve extraordinary things.**

2

THE WORLD'S MOST POWERFUL INDIVIDUAL

Great power comes easily to unique individuals. They are not necessarily out-of-the-ordinary people. Indeed, one of these individuals is very close to you . . .

In knowing ourselves to be unique, we possess the capacity for becoming conscious of the infinite. But only then!

Carl Jung

Have you ever met a truly powerful person?

Over the past few years I have met a great many people who are considered to be at the top of their tree. Among these were individuals of immense wealth, a few media magnates, international politicians, corporate leaders, sporting heroes, religious leaders, rock stars and actors, even a handful of gangsters.

Many of them oozed strength and authority. I can still recall how timid I sometimes felt in their presence. But on very few occasions did I sense real power.

I met a media magnate once. He was one of a hundred or so people on this earth who wield true global influence. Politicians and political parties in several countries vied for his favours. His decisions could influence financial markets. He could make things happen just as easily in the East as in the West. Yet he had no real power over the most basic elements of his life – he was a business automaton with no real existence outside the boardroom, and he was lonely.

I went on a rock tour once. The star of this tour was a man of immense wealth, admiration, and success far beyond his talent. He could go to one of a dozen countries and have thousands of devotees blindly follow his every suggestion. Yet he had no real power over the most basic elements of his life – he was unhappy and unfulfilled.

I met a high-ranking martial arts master once. He owned more than thirty academies in three cities, and had a financial interest in about the same number of successful restaurants. He boasted to me that extreme generosity could only come from someone who possessed unlimited power (meaning himself, I think). He was a man of great wealth and influence. Yet he had no power over the most basic element of his life – he was in a Hong Kong jail.

While not all the accomplished people I know are disconsolate or down, many of them do not possess the personal power that their worldly achievements would suggest. Because they do not have the power to alter their lives, or the direction of their lives, to accommodate their most basic needs.

How would it feel to discover you can easily attain such power?

The shift of power

The past millennium has been an interesting period for power. Just look at some of the major shifts that have taken place:

- the global expansion of major religions

- the glorification of science

- the advent of the Iron, Industrial, Technological and Information Ages

- the export of popular culture

- the growth of mass media and, with it, the concept of the 'global village'

- the rise and decline of social structures such as feudalism, socialism, despotism, feminism, capitalism, unionism, Puritanism, communism, colonialism, Bolshevism, Calvinism, fascism, globalism . . .

Interesting how so many of the above are '–isms' . . . collective ideals based around groups, trends, states and the common good (whatever that might be). It is a well-worn argument that we've reached a stage in history where selfishness has had its day, and our attention should be redirected towards the welfare of all humanity. But who gives *any of us* permission to speak for all humanity?

And, while I cannot profess to know what all humanity is thinking, I find it curious that almost all of these –isms are based on the concept that some individual thinks he or she knows what is best for the rest of us. And this 'knowledge' is usually imparted to us in some sort of prescriptive, 'either/or' framework. Don't you find it presumptuous that a person – invariably someone you've never met, probably never even heard of – presumes to know what's best for you?

So, what's the alternative?

I hesitate to suggest another –ism, such as individualism, with its overtones of selfishness and lack of compassion. So let's put aside the labels for a moment, and think of the characteristics of our ideal.

First of all, this ideal is steeped in respect for the power and uniqueness of each and every one of us. Secondly, there is the recognition that, along with this power, comes responsibility – responsibility to shape your own destiny, and the responsibility to use your accomplishments to make a difference with your life. Finally, and most importantly, this ideal is built around the notion that there is only one person in the universe who really knows what's best for you.

Yes, that's you.

At first, you might feel uncomfortable with this argument. Most people initially struggle to accept it – even as a possibility. Worse, many go through their entire lives without even contemplating it until it's too late.

This is understandable, since most of us have been brought up to defer to authority, assured that there is always someone who 'knows better' than we do – a parent, teacher, doctor, manager, priest, politician.

Yet, the older we get, and the more parents, teachers, doctors, managers, priests and politicians we actually encounter, the more convinced we become that they really don't know better at all. At least not when the issues concern us as individuals.

When it comes to matters of your health, for example, there is only one person in the universe who can keep you healthy, or cure you, or allow you to be cured. Just as there is only one person in the universe who knows, with any degree of certainty, whether you will be well or not. When it comes to matters of your soul or your spirit, there is only one person in the universe who can really tell you what is right, how you should think, or the course you should follow.

When it comes to matters of achievement, creativity, relationships, of peace of mind – anything that relates to you at all – there is only one person in the world who knows exactly what you should do, or what is best for you.

And that person is you.

Why you?

By any measure, you are a remarkable being. Even though you are but one of billions, on a planet that is one among billions, there is no other person in the universe quite like you. You are unique –

physiologically speaking, a miraculous achievement. Even though your entire life will account for no more than a micro-blip in time, you have an integral, irreplaceable role to play in the function and history of the universe. This is one fact that all the world's scientists and philosophers agree on:

The world would not be the same without you.

So while you may feel powerless to influence even the family next door, let alone events in distant galaxies, you are capable of the extra-ordinary. If you choose to, you can accomplish things that most of the world believes impossible. If you choose to, you can see God. If you choose to, you can attract wealth. If you choose to, you can heal your body using nothing but the power of your mind. You are capable of great feats of physical and emotional strength. You have access to the same depth of creativity that shaped the lives of Einstein, Van Gogh and Mozart. You can inspire with the simplest acts of generosity. You have the potential to make a difference, to make everything you do something of consequence.

Your first instinct may be to think I am writing about someone unrelated to you; someone with superhuman ambition, opportunities or capabilities. Far from it. The opportunities and capabilities I am referring to are well within the reach of *all* human beings; it's just that we have been trained to believe otherwise.

This is not an exaggeration: we have been *trained* from childhood to severely limit our potential. It is almost as if there were a conspiracy of teachers, spiritual advisers, management, governments, media and scientists.

Children are born with maximum potential, then spend the rest of their lives whittling it away. From their earliest days they can clearly hear colours and see sounds – until they are taught that colours cannot be heard, and sounds cannot be seen. From their earliest days their creativity is wondrous, and blossoms without limitation – until they learn that trees must be painted green, that sentences must never start with 'and', and that children should be seen and not heard. From their earliest days they can communicate with animals, absent friends and unseen beings – until they are forced to believe that this is impossible. From their earliest days their dreams are magical, and their ambitions know no bounds – until they learn that big dreams are not for people of their status, means or education.

And this process of censoring, editing, inhibiting and being taught what is impossible continues every day for the rest of their lives.

Is it sensible? No. Is it productive? Far from it. Nor does it make for happier, more contented or better people. All it means is that they will forever 'know their place' or 'know their limits' – as if these were benchmarks of character – and never try to rise above the station that society has defined for them.

Who knows best?

> *Some scientists claim that hydrogen, because it is so plentiful, is the basic building block of the universe. I dispute that. I say there is more stupidity than hydrogen, and that is the basic building block of the universe. Stupidity is replicating itself at an astonishing rate. It breeds easily and is self-financing.*
>
> Frank Zappa

Have you ever felt absolutely certain you were capable of doing something, only to be convinced by someone of much greater experience or authority that you were wrong?

Do you remember as a child when you painted bold pink stripes through the middle of your giraffe, and your teacher said: 'No, no, no, you're meant to paint *inside* the lines. And giraffes aren't pink.'

This is the role of authority: to ensure you conform and do not challenge the boundaries of what we accept as the norm.

Have you ever been in a situation where you felt absolutely certain you knew the answer to something, only to be convinced by someone more expert that you were completely wrong? This is one of the more common applications of expertise: proving others wrong.

Several years ago, when I started speaking about calm on talk shows and at universities, I discovered that expertise didn't always warrant the awe given to it. For every expert who sought to enlighten me with their wisdom, I'd encounter several who would try to silence me with it.

At first it was one simple academic pronouncement in relation to a comment I'd made about clinical hypnosis. 'That's not right!' he snapped.

'How is it not right?' I wondered.

'Because it's never been proven.'

I didn't think much about this until someone else used the same pronouncement. Then another, and another. Not only in relation to health and science, but to all aspects of life. You will notice this yourself: whenever you hear the words 'truth', 'proof' or 'reality' used more than once in a sentence, you can expect a good dose of arrogance to follow.

'There is *no* god.'

'How can you be sure?'

'Because you don't have any proof that there is.'

Does that sort of thinking bother you? It probably bothered people like da Vinci, Curie, Edison and Einstein, as well.

'Señor Columbus, everyone knows the earth is not round.'

'Mr Jenner, one cannot *prevent* smallpox.'

'Ms Earhart, everyone knows a woman's place is on the ground.'

'Mr Picasso, that's not the way to draw a woman's face.'

'Mr Dylan, that's no way to sing a ballad.'

One of the most difficult challenges in life is to reach beyond the expected, and perhaps to achieve something of consequence in the process.

Unfortunately, it is much easier to censor and to stifle than it is to create or to achieve. When it comes to areas outside the mainstream – such as in areas of human development that involve the mind and spirit – efforts to prove the other party wrong seem to increase exponentially. You see, expertise more often means knowing what is *not* true, rather than what is. (This is the nature of science. It is impossible to prove a scientific hypothesis true since no one can ever observe and verify all the possible evidence required to do so; it can only ever be proved that certain things are false.) One of history's greatest physicists, Niels Bohr, said: 'The opposite of a correct statement is a false statement. But the opposite of a profound truth may well be another profound truth.'

So who has the answers to life's questions?

I don't. You probably don't, either. But both of us can be relaxed about this because no-one has all the answers.

But you can have *access* to the answers that pertain to your life!

So, for the duration of this book, I want you to keep one thought firmly in mind: you have as much access to 'truth', 'proof' and 'reality' – particularly as it pertains to you – as any other human alive. Perhaps even more so.

Can you see what a powerful position that places you in?

Even more than the authorities

Great spirits often encounter violent opposition from mediocre minds.
Albert Einstein

From the earliest age, we have been trained to defer to higher authorities – parents, teachers, doctors, managers, scientists, priests, politicians. Often, we accept their assessments and opinions, without question, and apply them to our own lives. Yet, the question has to be asked, do these people know more about what is right for you than you do?

A good starting point would be to examine one of the cornerstones of our belief system: scientific proof adds certainty to life. Science and medicine have prospered over the decades because they have undertaken their research objectively, unemotionally and according to rigorous ethical standards. Ideally, then, scientific research would add proof and certainty to life.

It can't. Because while scientific research can often prove what *doesn't* work, it can only speculate on the probabilities of what *does*. (Most researchers will dispute this fact but, as we have discovered, it is impossible to verify *all* possible evidence to prove a scientific hypothesis.)

Take any 'big picture' topic, such as a human being. Even with the combined efforts of all the scientists in the world, we are incapable of fully understanding this single topic. For a start, research is carried out by human beings, which brings matters of intention, ambition and ego into play. Secondly, research budgets often dictate the priorities and choice of research projects. Thirdly, given the necessary funding and motivation, even the wildest biases can be given credibility. (You may have heard of the study that showed how smoking brings a net benefit to society – because smokers die younger, they reduce the strain placed on the medical system by an ageing population.) And, most important of all, the process of scientific discovery shows us that the closer we look at any given issue, the more we will find that cannot be explained; the more we learn, the less we know.

All we can ever be sure of is that probabilities exist. There is a probability that an atom exists, that a kilogram in New York weighs the same as a kilogram in Paris, that amino acids are the building blocks of life, that the universe began with the Big Bang . . . but there is also the possibility that these 'facts' are mere speculations.

What about medicine, then? Surely, with all the billions that are spent on medical research each year, the medical community would know more than you and I about what's best for your health. Most of us believe that modern medicine has our best interests at heart. After all, it is devoted to healing.

Oh, really?

In a broad sense, the nature of modern medicine is not concerned with healing so much as treating conditions or offering treatments. There is a fundamental difference between treating and healing.

Treatments are conducted in sterile, brightly lit environments where technology equates with efficiency. The focus is on the reversal of symptoms of illness. Usually, treatments are conducted without emotion, without examination of personal issues, and according to a strict time frame. In doing this, the doctor or technician instructs and the patient is meant to respond. This is why doctors seldom kill patients, but patients often 'fail to respond to treatment'. Extrapolating from this principle, if you die, you have only yourself to blame (for not responding). A subtle distinction, perhaps, but one worth bearing in mind next time you're feeling ill.

Healing, on the other hand, is quiet and reflective, seeking to instil balance and harmony in your life. Generally it occurs in relaxed, natural surroundings. Often it is ongoing, and is either self-administered or conducted in a cooperative environment. It is defined by a caring spirit, and a lack of urgency that allows for progressive change.(Modern medical practitioners *can* follow good healing practices, of course. And, I am pleased to report, more and more of them are doing so.)

I am not arguing the superiority of one approach over the other, merely highlighting the fact that when it comes to your health, *you* might have as much to offer as any medical authority. *You* might be the authority.

'But,' some say, 'our treatments work. You know very well that all medical procedures are clinically proven.' A powerful assumption. Indeed, one of the most potent weapons the medical profession employs against outsiders is the denunciation, 'It's not clinically proven'.

Ironically, very few medical procedures are clinically 'proven'. Most medical procedures have been developed according to a standard known as 'medical best practice' – often based on nothing more sophisticated than trial and error, albeit sometimes over many decades or even centuries. Medical best practice, though, is *not* proof.

'But surely,' you might argue, 'even if there are a few flaws now, medical services will keep on improving.' Only the dreamers believe that fantasy. In every country of the world, public medicine is at breaking point. The ever-increasing cost of delivering services, combined with the rising demands of an ageing and less robust population, means that a serious rethink needs to take place. The percentage of people suffering from medically induced conditions (through error, re-infection, contagion, drug or surgical side-effect) is also escalating at an alarming rate and, instead of there being an improvement in health services, there is a decline. What's more, it's going to get worse unless some form of attitudinal change takes place. The choices we have are:

(i)   spend more (difficult when in countries such as the United States health expenditure already accounts for 14 percent of the GDP);

(ii) restrict services to those with most resources (money), greatest need (the dangerously but not terminally ill), or greatest survival potential (young, female, non-smokers); or

(iii) promote preventative medicine so that individuals are urged to play a more meaningful role in their health, and so that the demands on hospitals and other medical services are lessened.

Naturally, I favour the last course. This is why much of what follows in this book is designed to enhance your wellbeing, and hopefully do away with the need for many medical services.

This brings us to the belief that alternative medicine is superior to conventional medicine in all but acute conditions. This is another increasingly popular, but potentially dangerous, assumption.

The concept of 'natural' therapies varies from person to person. Most believe it refers to mixtures and potions derived from natural, primarily botanical, sources. The belief is that, because of their naturalness, these substances function better than artificial equivalents. But just as there are some spectacular poisons (belladonna, botulin, strychnine) that come from natural sources, there are also many over-the-counter pharmaceuticals that come from natural sources. As for traditional medicine (acupuncture, Ayurvedic medicine, chiropractic, herbal medicine, homeopathy, naturopathy, osteopathy, traditional Chinese medicine), well, it can hardly be considered 'alternative' if up to 80 percent of the world's population still use it as their primary form of health care.

Most of the well-established alternative therapies have useful healing qualities – for some people. Some, like acupuncture, have such demonstrable benefits that they are now close to becoming mainstream medical practices. Others have so few demonstrable, reproducible and quantifiable benefits that they are often considered too esoteric to be taken seriously – yet they work for many people.

But are they superior? Sometimes – although their purpose is usually different to that of mainstream medicine. But it would be naïve to pretend that after so many decades of medical research, so much concentration by brilliant minds, so many billions of research dollars, that orthodox medicine does not have much to offer. It does.

In spite of all the advances in science, though, it is an inescapable fact that the modern world has been shaped more by spiritual yearnings and beliefs than by any other influence. You might assume that the one group of authorities you should be able to rely on to have the right answers are the more enlightened spiritual leaders.

Surely, simply by definition, the outcome of enlightenment would be a certain convergence of truths. Yet, there remains an extraordinary diversity in these areas. Do the various gods, each attracting millions of followers, have a hierarchy of relevance? Does the fact that you were born in Iran or China mean you are less likely to achieve salvation than someone born in Israel? Does someone born in India or Tibet have a greater chance of enlightenment than someone born in the United States? Is divine 'truth' really so sectarian than it excludes most of the world's spiritually aware population?

Fortunately, the one thing all religions and spiritual movements have in common is that their 'truth' cannot be observed or empirically analysed – it can only be experienced.

Such subjectivity means that one person has an extraordinary level of power when it comes to your spiritual development.

That person? You.

Objectivity vs subjectivity

If we take an *objective* (impartial) view of your life and capabilities, we might conclude that certain accomplishments are within your powers and others are beyond you. However, your *subjective* view (from within your mind and subject to your biases) may not be so restrictive.

Scientifically orientated folk have done a great job of elevating the importance of 'objectivity' in our view of life. They insist that objectivity should govern all fields of study. This can be an enormous limitation.

Anyone who insists on taking an objective view of history, for example, is destined for failure. As much as we would like to think the past has some sort of concrete dimension, we know that three people witnessing the same event only 30 minutes ago would describe it in three totally different ways; even if what they believe they saw was identical (which it would not be), their ways of describing it would vary.

Similarly, when you consider the human 'sciences', such as psychology, the quest for objectivity stands in the way of empathy and rapport. And, even in the physical sciences, quantum mechanics shows that simply by studying any particular event you become part of that event (to a measurable degree) – a participation that precludes objectivity.

When it comes to you and your life a subjective view is not only acceptable, it is essential!

You can do it easily

Ignorance is not the problem in the world. It's the things people 'know' that aren't so.

Will Rogers

I have pointed out the above variations in the nature of 'truth' and 'fact', not as an attempt to discredit any scientific, medical, academic, alternative, psychological or religious convictions, but as a way of illustrating that life is not as black and white as we have been led to believe.

Science and medicine do not have all the answers. There are great gaps of logic in New Age thinking. There is a great divergence of opinion over even the most fundamental issues in philosophy and spirituality. Experts hold opposing views about economics, the environment, politics – in fact, in almost all areas of life.

But in the midst of all this confusion, one truth stands out.

When it comes to determining what is truth and what is fact – as they pertain to you and your life – *you* play the major role.

With respect to the issues in your life, there is no-one on this planet who can tell you with any certainty: 'It can't be done.' Once you accept this, so much more becomes possible. In fact, *everything* becomes possible for you.

Once you believe you can achieve, heal, transform or transcend any thing or any situation, there is only one person in the universe who has the power to say whether or not it is achievable.

That is you.

There will always be those who say it can't be done. Many of them will be armed with 'facts', research and 'proof'. Some will try to batter you with expertise. They will cite superior understanding, insight or training. They might even be able to 'prove' it can't be done.

The world is full of experts and authorities who specialise in knowing not what is possible, but what is *im*possible.

They 'know' that it's impossible for you to overcome certain diseases, disabilities or mental states. They 'know' that untrained people from humble backgrounds cannot earn vast fortunes, or write bestsellers, or marry princesses, or paint masterpieces, or have high-octane successes from a calm state of mind. They 'know' such feats are impossible.

And if you do manage to accomplish the 'impossible', do they re-evaluate what they know? No. They dismiss your achievement as a fluke or aberration, as being statistically insignificant, or more often than not, as being simply delusionary. Those who accomplish these feats, and do so with ease, know achievements of this sort *are* aberrations. Of course they are. They go against the norm. But the norm exists only because we have been trained to believe we can never transcend it. We are constrained by our own belief systems.

Scientific experiments reveal this with monotonous regularity. When placebos are provided in controlled clinical experiments the recipients of such 'fake' medications often get better – simply because they believe they will get better. No big surprise there. Often, how-ever, these same people *also* develop the same side-effects as the group given the genuine medication. Because they believe these are the side-effects one gets. Belief not only plays a powerful role in healing, but in inducing illness as well. It's often observed in some of the less traditional cancer clinics that many, if not most, sufferers believe they know the 'cause' of their cancer.

What you believe is ultimately what you become. If you believe you will be well, happy, successful and popular, you will be well, happy, successful and popular. The converse also applies. It makes good sense, then, to make your beliefs start working for you.

It's time to free up your belief systems. It's time to recognise that some people do transcend the norm. You know from your own expe-rience that there are many who overcome the odds. They accomplish extraordinary things. They shrug off 'terminal' illnesses. They lead useful, contented lives. They have beautiful relationships. They find ways of being happy and successful at the same time. They make a difference.

You can become part of that group.

When you free up your belief systems, accomplishments of this nature not only become possible for you, they become accessible. By the end of this book you will know how to access them.

You have a choice

You can choose not to be bound by the limitations that you, and others on your behalf, have traditionally accepted. It is possible to sidestep these limitations and realise the vast potential that lies within every human being.

All it takes is a single decision and a few simple techniques.

Even though your life has been shaped by decades of conditioning, even if it is coloured by millions of years of evolution imprinted in your genes, you can alter the course of your existence with a subtle shift of attitude. You have the freedom and capacity to change, to achieve, to be calm. You have the freedom and capacity to make a difference.

But with this comes a responsibility. If you want the freedom and capacity to be able to make a difference in life, you must accept the responsibility for making a difference in life.

You can transfer this responsibility to someone else, of course; you can hand it over to a doctor, a professor, a priest, or an author like me. This book will still serve you well if you make that decision. But you must make the decision one way or the other.

Let's preview some of the choices that will unfold as this book progresses:

State	Belief	Choice
Happiness	All your life you've been told that happiness is something you'll have to strive for. Yet you also know that some people have the ability to just declare themselves happy.	You can take all the right steps, forever pursuing happiness . . . . . . or you can choose to be happy now.
Success and prosperity	You know that success comes to those who work long and hard at it, comforting themselves with the maxim, 'No pain, no gain'. Yet you also know that some people gain enormous achievements – quite naturally – without endless strain and effort.	You can plan for success, methodically following a certain course, hoping that you'll luck into it one day . . . . . . or you can choose to have it within the time frame you nominate.

State	Belief	Choice
Wisdom	From your earliest days you've been conditioned to believe that wisdom and enlightenment are the result of decades of searching, studying and dedication. Yet you also know that wisdom and enlightenment come to some people at very early ages.	You can pursue wisdom, incrementally, believing it will arrive some time in your old age . . . . . . or you can choose to have wisdom now
Peace of mind	Every day you hear what a stressful, competitive, amoral world we live in. How can anyone discover peace of mind in such chaos? Yet you also meet people who love every moment, and can't get enough of life.	You can carry the burdens of a bothersome age . . . . . . or you can choose to see the beauty and wonder in everything.
Healing	Scientific and medical research says certain illnesses, at certain stages, are incurable. When a leading specialist says you have one of these, you know there is no hope. Yet you also know that there are people who, contrary to the medical prognoses, overcome such illnesses and go on to lead normal lives.	You can follow the edicts of the medical authorities . . . . . . or you can choose to have good health.

I have spoken about your having the power and understanding to make decisions that are best for you. Most of this understanding already resides within you. You already have a vast reservoir of knowledge, memories, observations and intuition that you may have never even suspected existed, let alone used. It exists, though, and it can be used to start making a difference.

But, first, there is a decision to make. The decision to take control of your own life.

I urge you to pause now – just for 30 seconds or so – and give yourself permission to take control of your life. When you have done that, I'll show you how to do it.

The starting point is a specific state of inner peace that I call Deep Calm.

Soon you will know how to access it.

So far, you've discovered that:

- **Being calm is a choice.**

- **It is easy to become calm – at will.**

- **From this calm state you can achieve extraordinary things.**

- **You may be more in tune with 'truth' or reality – as it relates to you – than any scientist, teacher or medical authority.**

- **You already have the power and capacity to make a difference.**

The topics dealt with in this chapter are covered in much more detail on our web site at www.calmcentre.com/reader; the password you need is 'reader'.

3

AN IRON WILL AND A STEEL-TRAP MIND

*Most people derive their power from
the same place and a similar state.
Knowing how to access that place –
and that state – allows you to access
that power . . .*

Last night she dreamed she could fly again. A breathtakingly simple feat. All she had to do was concentrate and her feet would lift off the ground. Floating. And she could maintain this state indefinitely, increasing or decreasing altitude just by squeezing out a little extra willpower. Hovering. Soaring. Swooping. Detached.

Once a Perfect Woman, Paul Wilson

Have you ever dreamed you could fly? That, with nothing more than the application of willpower, or positive thoughts, you could conquer gravity? It's a common dream – and an illustration of the strength that some of us imagine willpower to have.

The 'will of iron' is a greatly admired attribute in our hard-working society. So much so that most of us believe willpower, or strength of personality, is all that's required to succeed, to triumph over adversity, to cure illness and to be happy. Yet so many strong-willed people fail, have marriage breakdowns, become ill, get depressed and die unhappy. How can this be?

Willpower – as you know it – will not enable you to achieve a single thing in life.

Willpower will not make you more creative when you need to be. Nor will it help you to overcome illness, run faster, jump higher, think more clearly, write better, calculate more accurately, or be a better leader. It can't even help you to relax.

You see evidence of this time and time again. Someone asks you to solve a problem, or make a line of poetry scan, or come up with a witty name for a speedboat, or recall an event from your distant past. If these do not come naturally or easily, you can apply all the willpower you possess to these tasks, and still lack inspiration. Similarly, if your tooth is aching, or you're feeling depressed, or your husband is cheating on you, you can apply all your willpower to lessening those feelings, and you will still experience the ache, the depression and the anger. Maybe even more so.

Willpower is nowhere near as powerful as you have been led to believe. It helps you to achieve very little in life. It is grossly overrated as a human attribute. (This does not mean I am advocating laziness or lack of discipline as an alternative.) 'Well then', you might say, 'perhaps it's a combination of willpower and *intellect* that is required. Surely intellect can help us achieve extraordinary things.'

Oh, really? Then, how come so many intellectually gifted people fail, have marriage breakdowns, become ill, get depressed and die unhappy?

We have been taught to revere intellect as if it were the defining characteristic of a human being. But it is not. Intellect is like willpower: it is an attribute that is valuable and possibly even desirable, but it will never enable you to make more of a difference in your life. Like willpower, it will not bring you any closer to achieving what you want just by applying it in increased quantities. After all, we have already determined that the more you know, the less you can be sure of.

So, if your inner resources of willpower and intellect aren't going to provide the answers in life, where can you look for inspiration?

The centre of the whole

The most beautiful thing we can experience is the mysterious. It is the source of all true art and science. He to whom the emotion is a stranger, who can no longer pause to wonder and stand rapt in awe is as good as dead: his eyes are closed.

Albert Einstein

What if I were to tell you that you possess a resource which, in matters that relate to you, is infinitely more powerful than the knowledge of all the scientists, psychologists, medical specialists and alternative therapists in the world? What if I were to tell you that you possess a resource that is significantly more powerful that the world's fastest super-computer?

You take this resource for granted. It's an aspect of your consciousness.

After spending many years researching the way the brain works, with all its complications and mysteries, it would be very easy to slip into a technical mode at this point.

I will avoid this.

There are aspects of consciousness that are beyond human comprehension, or at least this human's comprehension. As a result, they are subject to endless philosophical discussion. However, I will endeavour to simplify the more important elements.

Firstly, consciousness is usually defined as an ability to sense that you exist, and to be able to evaluate that experience in some way. You are conscious when you know some of what's going on around you, when you have a few memories you can recall, and when you have some degree of control over what you respond to and how you do it. You know you're conscious now because you're reading these words and hopefully understanding them. Easy.

But that's only one aspect of consciousness.

There are thousands – no, millions – of things going on within you and around you right now. At any given moment, you can focus your attention on one or, at most, a few of these. These will be the few than interest you, amuse you, intrigue you, stand out as different, or appeal to your emotions. What about all the rest?

Even though you are not aware of it, many of these millions of things are still impacting on your consciousness. For example, you're not consciously listening for cars looming up behind you, but as one approaches, your brain processes the information in such a way that you leap out of the way at precisely the right moment. *Subconsciously*, you could determine that danger was approaching, and consciously (or maybe subconsciously) decided to leap out of the way without really pausing to think about it.

Easy. You do it all the time.

Then there is yet another aspect of consciousness that you are not aware of at all. This is the *unconscious*. The reservoir of influences, biases, instincts and conditioned behaviours that we are seldom aware of – except that we know we behave in certain ways without really understanding why.

Fundamentally, your experience of the world is the product of three different levels of consciousness. Some say there are more, some say fewer, some say it's all a matter of attention. But broadly speaking the levels of consciousness are:

Conscious	Things that occupy your thoughts, attention and interest.
	Stimuli that you are aware of, and to some degree can control.
Subconscious	Information and stimuli that you take in without being aware of them.
	Experiences, observations and memories on the fringe of consciousness, which often just 'pop into your mind'.
	Memories, knowledge, sensations and emotions that can usually be accessed when required.
Unconscious	Deep-rooted biases, desires, memories, instincts and conditionings that influence your attitude and behaviour, usually without your being aware of it.
	Intuition, sixth sense, learned behaviours.

You're an expert on using the conscious part of your mind. You do it all the time, you depend on it, and you do it without ever thinking about it. Generally, you have little or no control over the subconscious or unconscious parts of your mind. Even though they represent by far the greatest part of your consciousness and your potential, they are seldom accessible to you. You've heard the comment that humans only use between five and ten percent of their brain's capacity? Now you know where that statistic comes from.

Much of what follows in this book is about learning to use the subconscious and unconscious parts of your mind to help you achieve the sorts of things you consciously 'know' can't be achieved.

Even though that may sound a little abstract or even difficult, you will find it's incredibly easy to accomplish – once you know how to access Deep Calm.

And, by the end of this book, you will know how.

Parts of the whole

Now we come to an aspect of consciousness that some find easier to accept because it relates to quantifiable, measurable or observable occurrences within the brain.

The brain is simple enough to understand. It's more pink matter than grey, it resides inside your head, and some people do more with it than others. It can do extraordinary things, not the least of which is actually thinking about itself.

There are three main parts to the brain: the brain stem, the cerebellum and the cerebrum. Each controls different functions. The brain stem is the most primitive part of the brain, controlling involuntary functions such as breathing, swallowing, digestion, sweating and the heartbeat. The cerebellum is responsible for the coordination of functions such as moving, walking, dexterity and balance. And the cerebrum controls sense perception and voluntary movement. The wrinkly bit on the top is the cerebral cortex which governs thinking, decision-making, learning, analysing, understanding and remembering.

The cerebrum is divided into two information-processing hemispheres, commonly known as the left brain and right brain. An intricate network of fibres connects them and allows information to pass from one side to the other.

Even though both hemispheres of the brain are functioning at all times, they do have separate roles: in other words, they process information independently, as well as in tandem. In the main, the left brain controls the right side of your body, while the right brain controls the left side of your body.

Each hemisphere has a distinct processing style. In most right-handed people, the primary attributes are as follows (in a left-handed person, those attributes may be reversed).

The left Essentially, the left hemisphere is associated with structured, reasoned, linear, analytical thought processes – the type of detailed thinking that is common, expected and highly regarded in the classroom or at work. It is the verbal side of the brain, and is associated with the 'masculine' and assertiveness.

Over the last three centuries, we have been trained to favour the functions associated with this side of the brain. A mistake!

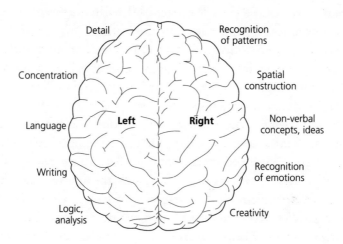

Detail

Recognition of patterns

Concentration

Spatial construction

Language   **Left**   **Right**

Non-verbal concepts, ideas

Writing

Recognition of emotions

Logic, analysis

Creativity

Left and right hemispheres of the brain

The right The right side of the brain is generally associated with the more imaginative, abstract, emotive or holistic processes. As a result, it is used less in structured, day-to-day activities. It is the visual side of the brain, and is associated with the 'feminine' and intuition.

Often habit, occupation, or self-perception fosters a dominant way of thinking in an individual. You sometimes hear of people being referred to as 'left-brain thinkers' (structured, detailed, analytical) – usually in a pejorative way by those who fancy themselves as more creative thinkers. Interestingly, you seldom hear the expression 'right-brain thinker' used in a pejorative sense.

Generally, we favour the analytical, left hemisphere of our brains in our thinking processes. This means we are governed by a close-up perspective on life rather than the wide-angle one normally associated with the right brain. Such thinking makes it difficult, if not impossible, to fully comprehend abstract explanations of life (especially at the quantum and universal levels). The only way of coming close to understanding such ideas is by being less rational and by adopting a more holistic way of thinking – utilising both hemispheres of the brain as one.

Left and right as one

Some psychologists refer to the left-brain function as the analyser – because most of the time it is occupied with analysis of data, conditions and practical information of this nature. This sort of activity is by nature restless and often intense. If you have to calculate, do a spreadsheet or research an issue, you automatically favour your left brain (analyser).

The right-brain function is known as the integrator, because its role is to take all of that analysed information and transform it into a seamless, holistic action – loving, singing, running, driving, healing – without your having to think about it. When you try to approach the performance side of life – athletics, exams, therapy, relationships, business, the arts – favouring the left-brain (analyser) style, you discover its limitations. Yet, if you adopt a right-brain approach, you have to think less about your performance and it becomes easier for you to succeed.

What we strive to achieve in meditation, creativity and the experience of harmony in life is synchrony between the two hemispheres. Indeed, this synchrony – where both hemispheres of the brain show an evenly distributed spread of activity – is clearly demonstrated by a brain scan of a person in a deep meditative state or experiencing peak creativity. So the sense of balance and harmony that is often reported during meditation is more than metaphorical: it is physiological.

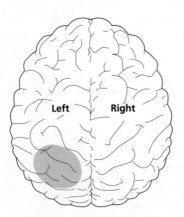

Normal daytime brain activity

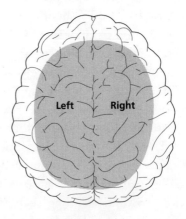

Meditative state

Deep Calm will help you achieve this synchrony. Moreover, it increases as you become more experienced.

Brainwaves

The brain is made up of billions of nerve cells called neurons. To accomplish even the simplest human task, millions of these neurons have to interconnect through a network of branches called dendrites, then act in unison to create an electrical impulse. The electrical impulse zaps down another branch (called an axon) and causes the release of a neurochemical which, in turn, activates other neurons.

The process of learning something, or doing something repetitively, begins to establish 'trails' known as neural pathways. The more you use these pathways, the more well-established they become, and the more 'engrained' the practice or way of thinking becomes. Imagine the neurons of the brain looking like a field of tall grass. Walk through it, from point A to B, and you leave a narrow trail. If you only go that way once, it will be soon be overgrown and forgotten. But walk along it 1000 times and you begin to wear a track – this is how neural pathways, or 'thought paths' become established. (Well-established neural pathways are the basis of habits. That is why undesirable habits are best overcome not by trying to eliminate them, but by establishing newer, more desirable ones.)

The electrical impulses by which the brain's neurons communicate are commonly referred to as brainwaves. These can be easily measured with an electroencephalograph (EEG) – which, although you probably don't own one, is a common enough machine. Electrodes are taped to the outside of a person's head, and leads from these are plugged into an EEG; then, as the person performs various mental functions, the associated electrical changes in the brain are recorded on a monitor or graph.

Every mental state you experience, every thought or emotion you have, is accompanied by a unique set of electrical impulses in the brain. And, as the left hemisphere of the brain usually reacts a little differently from the right, an EEG can be used to monitor each hemisphere separately.

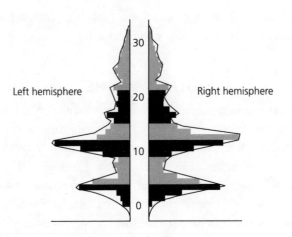

Left hemisphere   Right hemisphere

An example of an EEG readout

The brainwave frequencies that relate to different mental states are commonly grouped into bands. The first band was discovered in 1929. These were in the 7–12 Hz range and, probably because they were first to be discovered, were referred to as alpha frequencies. Subsequent discoveries revealed the beta range of frequencies (12–30 Hz), delta (0.5–3 Hz), theta (3–7 Hz), gamma (30–60 Hz) and lamda (60–120 Hz). Of these, only beta, alpha, theta and delta seem to relate to consciousness.

Before I go on to explain how this information can be used to transform the way you approach life, and what you can get out of it, let's examine these frequency bands more closely.

Beta, β 👁 👁 The brainwave state modern humans are most familiar with. This is your everyday, wide-awake, concentrating, thinking state. It dominates when your focus is on the outside world, and gets more intense as your stress levels rise. In the beta state, your creativity, intuition, emotions and even empathy are greatly suppressed.

Today, the beta state dominates for most of the day. Some say it was less dominant only 50 years ago (although measuring equipment has changed a little over this time, so it's difficult to be precise). Two centuries ago, it would probably have dominated even less, because there was more of a balance between stimulating and relaxing activities; today, our focus is almost entirely on stimulation – we even use stimulating activities (television, movies, music, parties) to 'relax'.

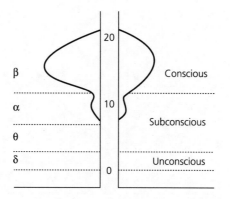

Normal waking state, beta-intense frequencies

To make this state a little more descriptive, I am going to refer to this state as beta-intense from now on. Because when your beta waves are most pronounced, you are feeling intense.

Alpha, α 👁 👁
Alpha waves rise, and will often be dominant, when you're relaxed yet alert – especially when you're daydreaming or fantasising. The beta frequencies will still be evident, depending on how much thinking you're doing at that moment.

The alpha state used to be known as the creative state. But having conducted many studies into the nature of creativity, and how to harness it, I can assure you the alpha state is *not* the creative state – though you could argue that it's much more conducive to creativity than the beta state.

Most of the research into the workings of the brain of the past 30 or 40 years has concentrated on this alpha state. Why? Because it was thought to be a meditative type state (it's not), and because it facilitated creativity (it doesn't). Probably, though, there was another reason it appealed to researchers: people can activate it quite easily, by means of a range of postures, expressions or thought processes.

From now on, I am going to refer to this state as alpha-relaxed.

I believe that the most important function of the alpha-relaxed state is as a 'go-between state'. To understand this, we need to look at the next two states – both of which operate at a subconscious or unconscious level.

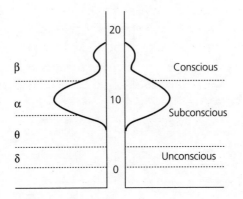

The relaxed but alert alpha-relaxed frequencies

Theta, θ 👁 👁   Theta waves are present in those beautiful, inspiring moments just before you drift off to sleep. Arthur Koestler referred to these moments in his book *Act of Creation:* 'The most fertile region [in the mind's inner landscape] seems to be the marshy shore between sleep and full awakening.'

When you have a flash of inspiration, or you sense something about a particular person or situation, or you experience a thought or feeling from the past, theta waves will be elevated. So, if there is such a state as the creative state, then it is this one – the theta state.

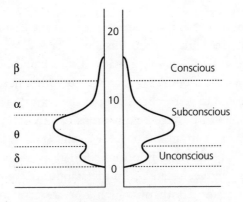

The theta-open frequencies

Many years ago, researchers began referring to the theta state as the 'yogic state' because Indian yogis could reproduce this state more or less at will. The theta state combines with alpha during meditation; ideally, these overwhelm the beta frequencies altogether.

From now on, I am going to refer to this state as theta-open, because at this level, your subconscious and unconscious begin to open up and reveal themselves to you.

Delta, δ

Delta waves dominate when you're asleep, and at the unconscious level. However, they also make their presence felt when you're wide awake. This is known as intuition. You will be familiar with the experience of saying the same thing at exactly the same time as someone close to you. Or 'sensing' something about another person without having any reasonable evidence that what you sense may be correct. On an intuitive or deeply empathetic level, you are in tune with these things but are not consciously aware of them. You just feel them. Intuitive or psychic types often have pronounced delta wave activity during their normal waking states.

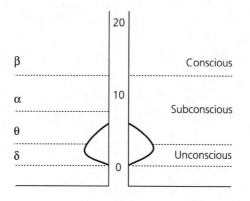

The sleepy delta-zzz frequencies

From now on, I am going to refer to this state as delta-zzz.

You are not normally aware of things that happen at the theta and delta levels. Occasionally you will have flashes of inspiration from these brainwave patterns, but they are difficult to produce at will.

The relaxed states

Alpha-relaxed waves are present when you're relaxed, but wide awake. As you move into deeper levels of relaxation, two things start to happen: beta-intense waves diminish; and theta-open waves rise. This is a deeply relaxed state – about as 'relaxed' as you can hope to be in everyday life without falling asleep and without using techniques like meditation to take you into deeper states.

While I use the word 'relaxed' to describe the state most commonly known as meditation, it is much more than relaxation. For a start, it is an altered state that falls outside the usual boundaries. Those who understand it, and practise it, appreciate it as the one state where they feel totally natural and at peace – where they are aware of infinitely more than is possible in a wide-awake beta-intense state or in a deeply relaxed (unconscious) delta-zzz state.

During meditation, beta waves are almost non-existent, alpha and theta waves are pronounced, and delta waves are also present. These proportions vary according to the type of meditation and the attitude of the person but, broadly speaking, this is how they look.

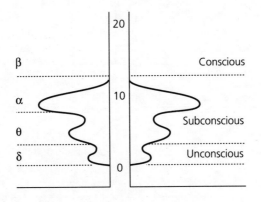

Brainwave pattern in meditation

Much of what is popularly written about alpha states and theta states is rubbish. The facts are:

- Most of the time, all types of frequencies are present, with one band dominant.

- The beta–dominant state (beta–intense) is the most common. Too much reliance on this state limits your potential in almost all fields in life. It limits your ability to be creative, to be intuitive, to access the vast reservoirs of memory, information, knowledge and wisdom that reside in your subconscious. These can only be reached through the theta and delta states.

- You cannot access the theta and delta levels from a beta state.

- When you are relaxing in the normal world, alpha waves dominate.

β	beta-intense 12–30 Hz	Work state	The manager	
		Concentration, analysis, worry	Logical, self-important	
		Outwardly focused	The 'editor' or 'censor'	
α	alpha-relaxed 7–12 Hz	Daydream state	The go-between	Conscious
		Relaxed, but alert		
		Bridge between conscious and subconscious	Moves information between states	
θ	theta-open 3–7 Hz	Yogic, meditative state		
		Creative	The dreamer	Subconscious
		In touch with subconscious		
δ	delta-zzz 0.5–3 Hz	Sleep state	Mysterious	
		In touch with unconscious, intuition, empathy, etc	The sleeper	Unconscious

The four major brainwave frequency bands

- One of the roles of the alpha-relaxed state is to form a bridge between your beta levels (conscious and fully aware of things) and your theta and delta levels (subconscious and unconscious).

If you want to go further than relaxation, if you want to go beyond the intellectual, creative and emotional boundaries that you normally live by, you need a connection between beta-intense (conscious) and theta/delta (subconscious/unconscious). Alpha-relaxed forms this bridge.

These brainwave patterns are not mystical. Just like your pulse or your heartbeat, they can be measured. There are many people like myself who, over the years, have researched how these frequencies relate to specific states of your existence. And, more importantly, *how you can manipulate these frequencies yourself, to bring about these states.*

This is known as neurofeedback, or biofeedback. Once you know how it works, you can control how you feel and how you react to certain situations. For example, you can ease yourself into a state of deep relaxation – just like that. Similarly, you can increase your creative ability of your athletic performance, or help to over-come illness – simply, easily and predictably.

These are not far-fetched ambitions. Almost every top athlete in the world knows how to use this ability. As do many people who have a professional need to be creative in their work. As do many medical practitioners who use it to assist in the treatment of life-threatening illnesses.

> *This is a real performance-enhancing ability which, whether they realise it or not, is used by almost all successful people.*

In the sections ahead, you will learn simple techniques that will allow you to access the deeper levels of your creativity and wisdom, so that you can achieve things you may once have considered impossible.

The whole

To know what is impenetrable to us really exists, manifesting itself as the highest wisdom and the most radiant beauty which our dull faculties can comprehend only in their more primitive forms – this knowledge, this feeling is at the centre of true religiousness.

Albert Einstein

Contained in this section is the key to using a specific state of inner calm to achieve whatever you believe is important in life – happiness, understanding, peace of mind, health, longevity, or worldly accomplishment.

Broadly speaking, there are two major ways of determining where you sit in regard to the rest of the universe. These two styles of thinking determine what direction you take – in health, business, sport, spiritual awareness, indeed in all of life's journeys. The style of thinking you will be most familiar with is the approach you've been trained to use since your first days of school; it dominates business, medicine, government and science, and has done so for hundreds of years. It's a structured, masculine, linear view of the world: a world of parts and pieces that function together as if the world were a sophisticated piece of machinery.

This way of understanding things is known as reductionism.

Reductionism When trying to understand any aspect of life using reductionist thinking, most of the effort is concentrated on under-standing the *parts* rather than the *whole* – whether the parts are organs of the human body, construction methods used to build the pyramids, or movements of Mozart's symphonies. These parts are then grouped into categories, in the hope of gaining a better understanding of the whole. Taking a reductionist view of the human body, for example, you identify groups of organs, tissues, cells and so on. If disease or malfunction appears in any one part, you focus your treatment on that particular part – either repairing, removing or replacing it.

With a few significant exceptions, most scientific research is conducted using reductionist techniques. So, too, is almost all orthodox medicine.

Why? Firstly, because that's the way we've been taught: it's logical, methodical and, frankly, it makes it much easier for someone to 'prove' their argument.

The second way of thinking is the opposite of this. It's known as holism.

Holism   Holism is a view of the world that focuses not on the parts, but on the 'whole'. It maintains that we can never understand the whole by analysing the parts; rather, we can best understand the parts by recognising the properties of the whole. Even though the word has only been around since 1926, holism as a concept has existed as a concept for thousands of years. It formed part of Hippocrates' original philosophy on healing. It is the essence of Taoism, as well as of Tibetan, Indian and Chinese Buddhism. And it plays a large role in many indigenous cultures.

Holism endeavours to take a 'big picture' perspective on all understanding – the person, the world, the universe. This is not always easy. Sometimes it's difficult to recognise exactly what the big picture is; how are we to know whether what we see is the 'whole' or just a fragment? Even highly trained scientists, philosophers and therapists have this difficulty. But there are ways, as you will discover later in this book.

How does holistic thinking manifest itself?

In relation to health, it recognises the wholeness of a person – a mind and spirit as well as a body. So, in matters of healing, your attitudes and belief systems are considered just as relevant to your wellness as any organ that may be troubling you. The literal meaning of the word heal is 'to make healthy or whole'. So holism and healing go hand in hand.

In science, a holistic approach recognises that the universe is one big undivided whole, in which everything is interconnected and of relevance. While this may be gaining acceptance in meteorology, sociology, biology and some of the more enlightened quarters of physics, such a principle is scorned in most other sciences. The detractors say that if we accept the chaotic nature of the universe, holism is meaningless. However, many of today's great thinkers are suggesting that the universe may have consciousness (as much evidence suggests), whereupon a holistic explanation of the nature of the universe makes a lot more sense. Even then, there is another barrier: holistic theories are difficult to 'prove'. They lack facts and precision. More challenging still, they require a different kind of perceptivity to accept and understand.

If you've been brought up in the reductionist tradition of thinking, your view of any aspect of life will probably be, 'seeing is believing'. If you'd been brought up in a holistic tradition of thinking, you would know that what you see is influenced by what you expect to see. Psychologists would agree with the latter. So, too, would all those physicists who accept that the intention of the researcher can have a direct influence on the outcome of an experiment.

This was beautifully demonstrated in 1905 when Albert Einstein was conducting experiments into the nature of light. Until then, light had been thought to exist as a continuous wave, but some of his experiments showed it to be made up of particles instead. Einstein's conclusion? If you go looking for particles, you discover that light is a particle; but, if you go looking for waves, you discover that light is a wave.

As you would expect, a conclusion like that threw a lot of spanners into the reductionist works of the scientific community and, more or less, prompted the birth of quantum physics. In the process, scientists were forced to accede to a preposterous-sounding theory called Heisenberg's Uncertainty Principle. According to this principle, when looking at pairs of physical properties dealing with space, time and energy, it is impossible to be accurate (more or less).

Doesn't that make you feel better? Imagine having to go to your boss or your professor with a conclusion like that! 'It's impossible to be accurate.'

Once again, we are faced with the possibility that you may be as in tune with the 'truth' or reality – as it pertains to you – as any scientist, economist, academic or medical authority.

Reductionism	Holism
parts	the whole
structured	creative
rational	intuitive
'prove it'	open
linear	non-linear
quantitative	qualitative
Western	Eastern
hierarchical	synergetic
opposite	complementary
categories	individuals
discrete	connected
future/past	now
precise	'fuzzy'
static	flowing
masculine	feminine
interventionist	self-correcting
single notes	harmony
mechanistic	humanistic

The two ways of thinking

What does all this mean to you?

Let's place these two ways of thinking in a more meaningful context. Say you've been complaining about a headache for two days.

Using a reductionist approach, your doctor will start 'diagnosing': you tell him about the troubled *part* (headache), then progressively provide more symptoms (sore throat and fever), until a picture emerges of a pre-defined *category* (flu). Your doctor diagnoses that you have the flu . . . because you have a number of symptoms. You are now expected to defer to the doctor's authority and be treated in the same way as everyone else in the 'flu' category. You may be offered antibiotics for your sore throat and aspirin for your headache – treating these *parts* as separate entities without due regard for the effect on the *whole* body.

You can see why such an approach is popular: if your sore throat and headache eventually go, the treatment is considered a success. Little matter that the flu returns a few weeks later, then you develop a candida infection as a side-effect of taking the antibiotics. Little matter that each time you go through this process, the antibiotics reduce your immunity to other illnesses, and the aspirin aggravates a peptic ulcer you didn't even know you had! So much for the reductionist approach.

The holistic approach is the antithesis of that.

For a start, the doctor or practitioner (if there's one involved) doesn't immediately start probing for symptoms, wondering what's wrong with you. Instead, they seek your guidance, your special knowledge of yourself in the context of the rest of your life. This includes your values and beliefs. In a spirit of cooperation, the practitioner leads you to modify or profit by this particular experience. Central to this process is the belief that you are not expected to be wholly ill or wholly well – because your wellbeing is a continuum of varying states.

You might decide that your headache is the result of a complex set of circumstances: your proximity to two sniffling children, who were in your range because you were staying at a friend's house because you had moved out of your family home, which you'd done because your husband became abusive after he was fired from work . . . and the stress of all this had caused your immune system to become run-down.

So, to modify this situation, you might seek counselling or a meditation course to help you adjust to your lifestyle changes. You might also take a herbal or homeopathic remedy to help your immune system return to normal. Oh, and you might even have a massage to relieve your headache.

The conclusion to this holistic process is that you might decide the headache was not a bad thing at all. It caused you to consider other factors in your life that needed balancing, so that your whole life could be improved.

Reductionism	Holism
concentrates on malfunctioning part	concentrates on whole person
diagnostic	intuitive
diseased organs	system imbalances
body orientated	body, mind and spirit orientated
Western	Eastern
categories of illness	an individual
either/or	continuum
static	flowing
interventionist	self-correcting
medical 'problems'	challenges to wellbeing
doctor the authority	doctor–patient team
patient the sufferer	patient the healer
cure	growth of self
body as machine	a human being

The two approaches to health

In reality, even a reductionist approach to medicine uses holistic principles sometimes. Similarly, holistic healing uses reductionist principles sometimes, such as when herbal or homeopathic remedies are prescribed to treat certain conditions. But when it comes to how you *feel* – that is, about feeling calm or tense, about feeling content or discontent, about feeling secure or insecure – you will find that a holistic perspective helps you feel calmer, more contented, more secure every time.

Every time.

The wider and more holistic your view, the more harmony, peace and space you will discover. Why? Probably because a holistic view requires more than mental effort. Because it involves more than just the mind, more than just the mind and body, you have to be able to *sense* it as well as conceive of it. The wide perspective leads to calm, while concentrating on the detail produces unrest.

You have unlimited creative potential

I have emphasised the importance of holistic thinking versus reductionist thinking for one simple reason: every self-made successful person I have ever met uses it.

Bear in mind I am speaking about major successes here – people who have made a difference not only in their own lives, but in the world around them. This includes every politician, businessperson, athlete, artist, academic and scientist who is calmly and deliberately making a difference. It includes every teacher, yogi, grand master, guru and cleric who is making a difference in their world. It also includes *most* of those I know who have overcome life-threatening illnesses.

It does not include artists who are discovered by others, people considered to be artistic or athletic phenomena, or people whose success comes from investment windfalls or privileged positions.

> *Every person who has calmly taken control of their lives and achieved things of significance – for themselves and the world around them – uses holistic principles to produce their success.*

Holistic ideals are not always easy to understand, at least not in an intellectual sense. Nor are they always easy to adhere to. If your kidneys are hurting, you might not care about the whole – you just want the pain to stop. If the kids in your neighbourhood are vandalising the local park, you may not care about the big picture – you just want the mayhem to stop. This probably also applies to the hole in the ozone layer, the money for this month's phone bill, and the unfair attitude your boss has been displaying of late.

But the big breakthroughs in your life – the ones that will really make a difference – will come from a holistic way of thinking. Now that you are aware of it, you will see more and more evidence of it as you go through life. This applies to:

- Meditation
- Diet
- Wellbeing
- Healing
- Mental health
- Music and the arts

- Understanding
- Decision-making
- Creativity
- Spirituality
- Sports
- Martial arts

Please don't fall into the trap of dismissing this as a New Age fad or a product of the frustration felt by those who feel powerless in the world as it stands. I can assure you that many powerful people use exactly this way of thinking. This is why so many philosophers, scientists, healing practitioners, teachers, as well as artists and businesspeople are embracing holistic principles as the *only* way of thinking that doesn't stifle your creative potential. This is the potential that will allow you to achieve the things that will make a difference.

Making a difference

If you're wondering why I keep referring to 'making a difference', it's because making a difference is the price you are expected to pay for the benefits you will gain from applying the techniques later in this book. This is not some rule I invented; it is a principle of focus.

If your focus is solely on yourself and your achievements, you will find it difficult to realise the beyond-the-norm accomplishments I keep referring to. This is not a matter of justice or karma (or perhaps it is!), but rather a matter of holism. When you adopt a holistic focus in what you do, you will see yourself as part of a much larger scheme. Being able to see yourself in this context is what enables you to rise above the singular limitations you have been taught to accept.

Holistic perception

Although it's covered in greater detail later in this book, this simple experiment will give you an inkling of what it's like to be able to perceive the world more holistically. (I must emphasise that this demonstration is only *partially* holistic – if you can tolerate such a contradiction in terms.)

Have you ever driven a car quickly?

You sit in the driver's seat, decide to drive to the stop lights around the next corner, then take off with your wheels spinning. While you're speeding down the street, you perform a thousand tiny actions. You control the car's speed with the accelerator pedal, touch the brake as you near the corner, scan every driveway along the street to check that no car is about to reverse into your path, listen to the revs of the engine to check that you're in the right gear, listen out for police sirens, and decide when you're going to hit the brakes so that you come to a halt before reaching the pedestrian crossing at the stop sign.

To do this successfully, you need to have a holistic perspective of the actual driving of the car. Because if you narrow your focus to any one of the activities involved – such as exactly how far to lift your foot off the accelerator pedal as you head into the corner, or on the driveway on the left as you go past – you'll have an accident. (To really view this action holistically, you would need to further broaden your perspective. You would need to take into account the social impact of someone speeding through a suburban street, risking the lives of the drivers and bike-riding children in that neighbourhood. You might also take into account that the world is so overpopulated as it is that the loss of a few inhabitants might be a positive outcome. Taking it further . . . well, you see how far this can go.)

The point I am endeavouring to make is that a narrow perspective limits your progress in life.

Here's something you can try right now. Somewhere in the room you are in is something that generates noise. Perhaps it's the fluorescent light tube, the buzz of your air conditioner, the whirr of the hard drive in your computer, or the breathing of the person beside you. Turn and look at the source of that sound. What can you hear? Not much. Okay, now narrow your focus. Look at that object or person. Look closer and closer. Really concentrate. What can you hear? Even less.

If you want to hear more, and at the same time become aware of other things going on around you – how the air conditioner vibrates or how the person's shoulders rise and fall as they breathe – all you have to do is stop concentrating. And widen your perspective.

The way you do this is with your eyes.

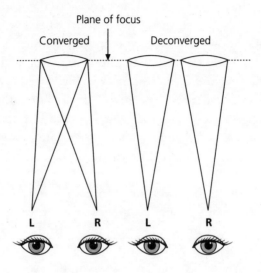

Convergence and deconvergence

Normally your eyes *converge* at the point where they focus; this is what enables you to perceive depth and dimension.

If you allow your eyes to *deconverge*, their plane of focus remains the same, but each eye continues to look straight ahead.

If you allow your eyes to deconverge, you will suddenly become aware of much more going on around you. Not only will you have access to more visual information, but you will hear more or feel more, according to where you focus your thoughts.

Deconvergence is simple to achieve. All you have to do is widen your peripheral vision as much as possible, without moving your eyes. Keeping your gaze fixed directly ahead, allow your peripheral vision to widen to take in more of the room around you.

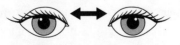

The wider your visual perspective, the more you will take in through your other senses.

This is a very powerful little piece of knowledge. You can apply it in so many different ways:

- If you want to really hear what someone is saying, and extract more of the nuances from their words, simply allow your eyes to deconverge and let all your senses go to work.

- If you want to really take in what another person is doing, allow your eyes to deconverge and let all your senses go to work.

- If you want to perform well an action that you have already done many times – a golf swing or dance movement – let your eyes deconverge and allow your other senses to play a role.

Is the simple act of widening your peripheral vision tantamount to taking a more holistic view?

Strictly speaking, a holistic view requires considerably more effort than this. But as a first step, it can't be beaten.

Try it. You'll see that it works.

The centre

As we have discussed, it can be difficult to maintain a holistic view of yourself and the universe. Are you part of it or outside of it? Are you at the left edge, or the bottom quarter, or the top right quartile? How do you know where you stand in relation to the 'whole'? Here's a simple exercise that could alter the way you see yourself in relation to the rest of the world. And thus put the whole notion of holism into perspective.

You know that the universe, by definition, is infinite.

So, if you look straight upwards, the distance between you and the edge of the universe is infinity (∞). Now, if you look straight downwards, past your feet, through the earth, you'll find the distance between you and the other edge of the universe is exactly the same – infinity (∞). And it doesn't matter which way you turn, the distance between you and the edge of the universe remains unchanged – infinity (∞).

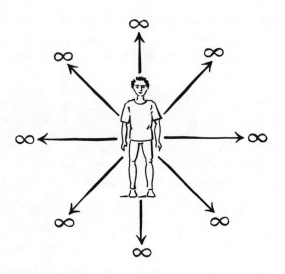

Guess where that places you.

Exactly. Smack in the centre of the universe. At this very moment, the person standing at the very centre of the universe is none other than you. So, next time someone says you act like the universe revolves around you, they're right! (Of course, there has to be an infinite number of centres of the universe to accommodate this.)

There's something very powerful and mystical about the centre. The most stable part of a solid sphere is the centre. The most stable position in any static object is the centre of gravity. The most powerful place from which to direct action in martial arts is from the centre.

> *Perhaps then it is not so surprising that the most serene and satisfying place to visit during meditation is the centre. Or somewhere you perceive to be the centre.*

This is why actors and singers, in the moments before a great performance, seek to 'centre' themselves – quietly, reflectively and alone. This is why athletes stand quietly in the moments before the starting pistol is fired, trying to centre their emotions and energies. Likewise musicians, painters and therapists all seek to find their centre before attempting a feat. This is why warriors strive to centre themselves before battle, as do surgeons preparing for a challenging operation. And it is also why 'the centre' features so prominently in spiritual and meditation traditions, particularly in its iconography.

The first major spiritual or mystical 'centre' that we know of was Stonehenge. Originally constructed about 3100 BC, it was rebuilt in 2100 BC, 1550 BC and again in 1100 BC.

The centre also featured in hieroglyphics used in the Egyptian pyramids as early as 3000 BC.

The enneagram used by pre-Islamic Sufis had many variations, all featuring nine points equidistant from one central point. It symbolised universal harmony and the journey into the self.

The mandala of Hindu and Buddhist traditions is a graphic representation of the universe – a focal point for its forces and energies, accessed through meditation.

Hindu and Buddhist chakras (Sanskrit for 'wheels'), which represent psychic-energy centres of the body, are usually depicted as wheels of energy.

The Taoist Yin–Yang graphic illustrates the balance of opposites in the universe, and their integrity: male/female, night/day, black/white, wind/water.

Christianity has adopted many ancient graphics based on a concept of the centre. This pagan monogram was adopted by the first Christian Roman emperor, Constantine. It is still used today.

Little wonder, then, that so many cultures and teaching traditions sought out this 'centre'.

Today, most of the Western world would consider their centre to be somewhere inside their head. In my earlier book, *The Calm Technique*, I located it in the hypothalamus, at the base of the brain – arbitrarily, I confess. According to the Aristotelean tradition, the human psychic centre is located at the heart, the seat of feeling, love and thought. In Taoist tradition, it resides at the tan tien, three finger widths below the navel. And in Hindu and Buddhist tradition, it tends to move about the place, residing in any one of seven different centres (chakras) throughout the body.

In all cases, though, the launching point of your psychic, emotional and spiritual essence is perceived as a 'centre' – so much so that it enjoys an almost mystical significance in the pursuit of human accomplishment. You have probably already sensed this yourself. On those occasions when you have felt complete, powerful, inspired, or simply at peace with the world, you almost surely recognised this as a deeply 'centred' state.

The precise location of your centre is not a matter of importance. What is important is that you intuitively associate some place within yourself with feelings of strength and ability. When you know how to find this place, and to access it at will, you have an extraordinarily powerful resource at your disposal.

Finding your centre

All my early research into meditation and calming techniques was focused on the East. Time and time again, the topic of finding your centre would arise.

When you stand in the unspoilt mountains of Tibet, a million miles from television and road rage, it is easy to feel you are at the centre of an extraordinary world. When you sail up the Yangtse River, gasping at the monoliths hewn from the rocky banks of the river and at the hidden Taoist monasteries that have stood for 1000 years or more, it's easy to believe you have arrived at the centre. So, too, when you stand on the remote slopes of Mount Abu in Rajasthan, with the smell of incense on the breeze and 3000 of years of tradition vested in the meditation teachings revealed to you that morning, it's impossible not to believe you are at the centre of the universe.

Then you go back to the city. And the traffic. And your television set and the office. Where is your centre now?

Where indeed?

I wrestled with this issue for many years. While it's easy for me – as an author – to encourage people to find the 'centre within', the reality is that this is a difficult task for people involved in busy lives. It was not until an event on New Year's Day 1989 that I finally understood exactly where to look for it.

This time it was not a research study. After a hard year, I'd gone to a remote island, just 30 minutes' boat ride off the coast of Noumea in the South Pacific, with the intention of editing a manuscript. You've never seen such a minuscule resort: 600 metres at its longest, it rose just 3 metres out of calm seas at its highest point. White sands. Tranquil. The shoreline was dotted with twenty small stone cottages hidden among the palm trees. By any criterion, this was an idyllic peaceful place. And relatively inexpensive at this time of year because, as I was soon to discover, it was the peak of the typhoon season.

In the past, the island residents had been evacuated during typhoons by the French Navy, based only half an hour away. However, Typhoon Delilah took an unexpected turn and, before the navy could even leave the port, high winds and rough seas washed away any thought of rescue. At the best of times, a typhoon is a menacing thing. If you're located on a tiny island that's capable of being totally submerged by a storm surge, this menace assumes a new dimension. This possibility was being openly canvassed by resort staff.

The central resort building of the island was designated as the gathering point. As fifty Japanese tourists were also stranded and the lack of English was intensifying the drama, my wife and I were given permission to retreat to our tiny stone cottage at the farthermost point of the island; we were assured by the resort management that it was as 'safe' as the central resort building and, if evacuation became possible, we would be advised.

I had experienced moderate cyclones as a child, and so believed I had an idea of what to expect. But the cyclones of my childhood were inland; the prospect of enduring one on a sandy speck in the middle of the South Pacific was quite something else.

I can't recall whether the build-up lasted 2 or 4 hours, but as night fell, the palms were bending to creaking point and the winds made it impossible to venture outside the tiny cottage. Our electricity had been severed, but coloured lights from the central building were still visible at times through the rain. Then they were gone. The island was in darkness. It's remarkable how much you can see in the moments before total darkness descends. The palms were bending, debris was swirling between them, but the sense of having survived was strong. My wife now felt relaxed enough to sleep. I was wide awake with the thought that, although the experience had been frightening, we were stronger for having survived it.

No sooner had I indulged in this self-congratulation than we discovered that Typhoon Delilah had not yet arrived. It arrived with such violence and noise that I could no longer even sense my thumping heart. Now the winds were so severe that the air seemed to be sucked from the room. Breathing was no longer automatic; you had to work on each breath. So much wind and air, yet so hard to get it into your lungs. That was not the worst of our fears. Each time water seeped into the blackened room, imagination insisted it was caused by rising sea levels rather than driving rain. And, even though the stone walls were a foot thick, I swear I could feel them creaking.

Then there was quiet. Not a normal quiet, but something mysterious and 'missing'. No wind. No sound of waves, birds or people. It was as if someone had muted the TV set. Now there was air in the room. We could breathe. We had survived!

This was only the eye of Typhoon Delilah: Act 2 was about to begin.

By morning, it had passed. The feared storm surge never materialised. The island was a shattered mess: it was strewn with building materials and broken trees; umbrella shafts had been driven into stone walls; even parts of the swimming pool had been smashed. Winds had been measured at 220 kilometres per hour, the maximum that local measuring equipment could register. We had been battered by a Category 4 typhoon, and I had lived to write this book. But the point of this story is not survival. It is the realisation that took place in the middle of the night when Delilah was at its peak.

When you are in the grip of a natural force so spectacular and awesome that it literally sucks your breath away; when you have plenty of time to contemplate your imminent death and there is not a thing you can do to avert it; and when you are known the world over as an authority on calm, it's time to put your preachings to the test.

Strangely, it was not fear that I had to contend with. The surreal nature of what was happening tended to preclude that. No, it was more a sense of panic (a combination of airlessness, darkness, noise and uncertainty) and physical stress. All of the calming skills I had acquired, up until that moment, had been formulated in the most beautiful, tranquil environments – often in exotic parts of the world. Now, faced with darkness and rising sea levels, they did not mean a thing. Yet, as the first half of the storm passed – in the moments of comparative quiet and stillness which signalled that the eye of the typhoon was passing right over us – I developed my first real insight into the nature of calm.

Journey to the centre

It is one thing to talk about the centre and what a restful and powerful place it is, but it is another thing entirely to have access to it.

Deep down, you are probably aware of what a wonderful state exists there. Most people know this intuitively. If you stop and think for a moment about where your centre is, or where it might be, you will find that your body begins to relax. In the first instance, that's all you have to do – think about where your centre is – for your body to begin to relax. Knowing this, then, is the first step to experiencing it.

Following are three different ways of 'centring' yourself, of moving to that inner state of calm, no matter what is going on in the world around you. When you reach this state – even if it is only for a few minutes – you will discover great peace and harmony, and clarity of mind. These techniques require only minimal time and effort to perfect. They are a good starting point for any of the calming techniques that appear later in this book.

Centring #1 Whatever you are doing, whatever is going on around you, just pause for a second and turn your attention to your breathing.

Just be aware of how each breath goes, slowly and deeply, to a restful place inside you. Be aware of this breath. Be aware of how relaxed it helps you to feel. That's all you have to do. A minute of this and you will feel like a new, calm person.

Centring #2 At any time of the day or night, imagine your body being filled with a powerful bright light. Although the light warms you, it would be invisible to an onlooker. Now, imagine that light growing in intensity until you begin to radiate its warmth and glow. The more you can feel yourself radiating this light, the more relaxed you will become.

Centring #3 Much of your energy – both psychic and physical – exists outside your body. Imagine fields of this energy surrounding you at this moment. With each breath you take, imagine this energy being drawn back into your body, coming to rest at your calm centre.

Even though these three exercises are very basic, each of them has the ability to instil a sense of calm and peace simply by turning your attention to the centre – by helping you to become aware of the fact that you *have* a calm centre. Being aware of this feeling provides you with a powerful resource for what is about to follow.

Looking in, looking out

The centring that we strive for in meditation, theatre or martial arts is usually a process of focusing inwards, sometimes as though we were external observers, until we reach – or at least sense – our centre. This is an introverted process. And, as with all introversion, it has its drawbacks.

If you have not done the years of training (bearing in mind that 20 years of meditation practice is normally required to become 'experienced'), you'll need great powers of concentration in order to achieve this.

You might be able to imagine how difficult it would be to con-centrate – to ignore the outside world and focus inwards – when the wind is screaming past your cottage at 220 kilometres per hour, you can't get air in your lungs, and you fear the storm tide could rise out of the darkness and swamp you at any moment. Try going inwards to find your centre then!

Yet, if your *starting point* is the centre – if you begin with the cognition of yourself at the centre and concentrate on looking outwards – you quickly find yourself in a very powerful position. Because you feel more able to deal with adverse forces if you are at the centre of the maelstrom – where comparative stillness prevails – rather than somewhere towards the edge, where you can't be sure which way it's going to turn next. You get a better idea of the music's melody and harmony when you are at the centre of the choir rather than half way along on the left. A large crowd is less daunting when you're at its centre rather than when it's approaching. Less energy is required to remain in the centre of a whirlpool rather than at the edge (not that you'd want to). In martial arts, you are in a more stable position when your opponent circles you, rather than when you circle your opponent.

Balance and harmony exist in the centre. Being able to go to your centre – at will – is the way for you to find balance and harmony in your life, no matter what is going on around you. It is vital that we have this ability, because there is no escaping the fact that we live in an increasingly tumultuous world.

Admittedly, I am referring to a subtle experience: a feeling or a perception more than a process. But once you have explored the centring techniques later in this book, you will find that this perspective is quite easy to attain. Then you will be able to go to your centre no matter what is going on in the world around you.

The experience of NOW

When you study martial arts, you are told that all strength and dexterity comes from being physically 'centred'. You are taught that centring the mind is the first step towards centring the body. For this reason, some martial arts use meditation not as a way of enriching the human experience, but as a way of reaching a more centred physical state. In many kung fu schools, for example, you will be told that the only way to be truly centred is to be in NOW, this present moment. If you think forward 30 seconds, you are no longer in the present, but are thinking of the future; similarly, if you wonder whether the move you just made was the correct one, you are no longer in the present, but in the past. This has a demonstrable weakening effect on you.

In case you think I'm being a little theoretical or abstract here, you can try this experiment for yourself. Place yourself in a physical position where you are finely balanced. Try standing on one leg, for instance. While you're in balance, something will be happening. You will be totally aware of the experience. All your senses will be heightened, but you will not be concentrating on any one of them. If you think about the precise placement of your foot, for example, you will overbalance. If you think about the top of your head, or the tip of your nose, or the point of your elbow, you will overbalance. You will only remain balanced as long as you are open to the total experience, not to any particular aspect of it. A holistic perspective on the experience, you might say. So far, that's easy to accept. You can put it to the test yourself and discover the importance of maintaining this perspective. But there's more.

You can only remain in this centred, finely balanced state if your experience is locked into the present. NOW. If you think ahead 30 seconds, wondering what your next move will be, you will overbalance. Similarly, the moment you think back 30 seconds, wondering if you completed a certain move the correct way, you will overbalance. Your balance depends on being centred in this very moment, now. The moment you think about the future or the past, your balance is upset.

Try it. This is a very revealing experiment – and one that leads to an understanding that martial arts students spend years trying to master. When you are physically centred, you are powerful. To be physically centred, you must be mentally centred. To be mentally centred, you cannot think about the experience (which turns it into an observation of the past), you can only experience it. To be mentally centred, you cannot think about the future or the past at all.

The only thing in life that is real is this very moment. NOW. It has no meaning; it is pure experience. When you are familiar with the practice of meditation, this is something you become aware of: there really is no beginning, no end, no past, no future – just the pure experience of now. When you are centred and experiencing this very instant, the past has no existence; it is just a thought. So, too, with the future. (There will be people who've had horrific experiences in the past who will write to me insisting that they are the products of these experiences, and that it is callous of me to say the past does not exist. Please be assured I have been through these arguments, as well as the usual space–time continuum arguments, yet I stand by this timeless assertion: when you can exist in the present, the past does not exist for you.)

Practise this experience of simply being in the moment – without analysis, without expectation – and you will be surprised at what you discover about yourself, and how wonderful life can be. Pure experience. An absolutely centred state. The experience of NOW.

There is a way of enabling this. But first, we must understand how we perceive time. At the Calm Centre (see page 98) we conducted a group of experiments to learn how people structured their vision of time, and whether these visions related to how relaxed, tense, optimistic or pessimistic they were. Broadly speaking, our results indicated that time perceptions varied, depending on a range of factors. These include occupation, personality and, unsurprisingly, age. (Please bear in mind that I am using generalisations to illustrate a technique, not to analyse personalities.)

If you look at the diagram over the page, the horizontal line represents time. Whether it represents 3 months or 30 years is not important (it varies from person to person); the past/future orientation is what interests us.

A past orientation (a) is common among older people. This is not surprising since it is representative of the investment such a person has made in their life – most has gone before, and planning is not such a feature any more. This orientation was also seen in most academics and many writers, and was common among those who prided themselves on their knowledge and learning. The past orientation did not specifically relate to either calm or tense feelings. However, people with this orientation often feared change and tended to have a pessimistic outlook. Also, this group was the only one in which emotions such as regret and guilt featured.

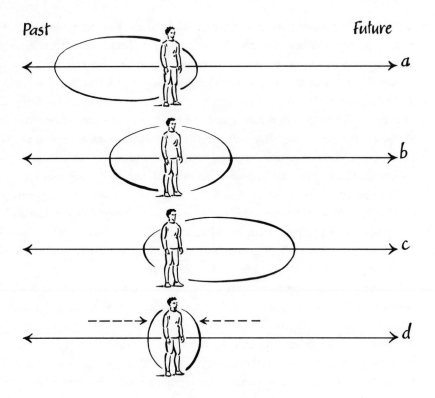

Perceptions of time

Those with a past/future orientation (b), were the most numerous. Their overriding perception of time was that there was 'so much to do, so little time to do it'. This group mostly featured people aged between 20 and 40. Primarily, their focus was on the day-to-day. And, even when they were planning for the future or analysing the past, their focus was on what was happening in their lives at that moment. 'Survival' is the word that springs to mind. This was the most highly stressed group (their assessment). It was also the most overwhelmed (their assessment).

The third group (c) were those with a future orientation. Made up of people of all ages, this group was dominated by the risk-averse, the dreamers and the creative. It was curious that risk-averse and creative people should feature in the same group since their behaviour was so different. The risk-averse concentrated on preserving what they had, and being on the lookout for problems that might arise in the future.

Creative people and dreamers tended to live in their imagination, planning things that might occur sometime in the future. Interestingly, this group reported the most optimistic and the most anxious feelings (often within the same person). I suppose this is understandable, since both of those feelings are based on the future. How did they feature on the calm/tense scale? Neither one way nor the other. Although creative people and dreamers did show a resilience to setback that neither the risk-averse nor those in (a) and (b) did.

This brings us to the last group (d), those whose focus was on NOW, the present. Unlike the others, this was not a well-defined group. Some of those in this group were not great role models: unemployed surfers, drop-outs, and others who could be described as less responsible, possibly even amoral. However this group also featured a range of people who possessed extreme human abilities – martial artists, long-term meditators, yogis, artists and so on. These people had the rare ability to live in the present, or at least to perceive themselves as living in the present, for much of their day. Generally, this is a matter of focus and concentration. When you can fully occupy yourself with one particular activity – regardless of what that activity may be – you discover the experience of NOW. When you can do this, becoming centred is much easier.

But there is another way that you can discover this NOW experience. All it takes is a simple adjustment in your imagination.

- Sit quietly for a few minutes, listening to the sound of your relaxed breathing.

- Tell yourself you have all the time in the world.

- Close your eyes and imagine that time stretches out in front of you and behind you.

- Look ahead some time into the future – a few hours away or tomorrow – and imagine it is in front of you. It doesn't matter what you can see, as long as you get a feeling for what the future is like.

- When you are comfortable with this, try looking back into your past. Imagine it is behind you. Once again, it doesn't matter what you can see, as long as you get a feeling for what the past is like.

- Now, in your imagination, gradually draw the future towards you until you can feel it becoming part of your present experience. At the same time, imagine drawing the past towards you until it, too, is part of your present. When these two feelings meet, you will have an experience of being in the present.

- Make a note of that feeling. Enjoy it. Stay with it for as long as you can. Once you become familiar and comfortable with this, it's amazing how quickly you can bring back that feeling . . . and so become calm and centred at will.

The nature of calm

One of the most surprisingly calm people I ever met was a boxer, a young Russian named Kostya Tszyu. Not only was he one of the youngest ever captains of the Russian Olympic boxing team, but he went on to become a world champion and to gain a reputation as one of the most powerful boxers of his weight division. Yet, in spite of the aggression and violence that is expected of him when he steps into the ring, he is an extraordinarily calm man. Peaceful. Moreover, he maintains that sense of calm for the duration of each bout. According to Tszyu, this state enables his most powerful feats.

This principle applies to almost every endeavour in life where you seek to rise above the norm. The greatest achievements come from a centred state of calm (a sense of inner calm).

Now, let's look at how you can achieve it.

So far, you've discovered that:

- Being calm is a choice.

- It is easy to become calm – at will.

- From this calm state you can achieve extraordinary things.

- You already have the power and capacity to make a difference.

- Willpower will not enable you to achieve a single thing in life.

- Calm and achievement are easier to gain when approached holistically.

- Your greatest power and your maximum potential come from your calm centre.

- You are totally centred when you exist in the moment – NOW.

4

THE CALM CENTRE'S NINE MENTAL POWERS

At this very instant you possess nine extraordinary powers. The following section will show you where to look for them . . .

I belong to a kind of 'calm think tank' called the Calm Centre. It's a loose collaboration of researchers, psychologists, natural therapists, writers and artists of various persuasions whose primary focus is to develop new ways to spread calm. Individually we have spent many years exploring why people act the way they do, think the way they do and, in particular, how they succumb to, or rise above, the limitations that they and others set for them.

What follows is a summary of our conclusions. They have been formulated as a set of principles for using the mind to effect change. These became the focus of a number of speeches, challenges and debates throughout the 1980s. Some of the discussions prompted us to add to the list, a couple of the principles have been modified, but overall the list remains more or less intact.

When you can influence the way you think and behave, you can influence the direction of your life.

When you choose to use the power of your mind to effect positive change – in terms of psychology, self-improvement, health and performance – there are nine principles that apply. These we now call the Calm Centre's Nine Mental Powers:

1. The Power of Choice

2. The Power of Calm

3. The Power of Substitution

4. The Power of the Subconscious

5. The Power of Emotion

6. The Power of Imagination

7. The Power of Repetition

8. The Power of Focus

9. The Power of NOW

These powers or principles are so central to achieving peace, prosperity and wellbeing, that I have devoted this entire chapter to them.

Read through them. Get a 'feel' for them. Because they underpin all the techniques and strategies this book contains.

1. The Power of Choice

Making a conscious choice to follow one direction in preference to another is an act that falls within all our capabilities. Even though it may sometimes take a change of perspective or an injection of creativity for you to recognise the fact, you always have choices.

You *can* change. You *can* change the way you think. You *can* change childhood conditioning. You *can* change your habits (yes, all habits). You *can* change your beliefs. You *can* change the way you behave.

Recognising this is the first step in making it happen.

2. The Power of Calm

If there is one principle that emerges over and over again throughout this book, it is this: the greatest achievements come from a calm state of mind, or a sense of inner calm. And nowhere is this more true than in the processes of the mind – in understanding, remembering, creativity, emotion, intuition, rapport, communication, you name it.

> *In matters of the mind, the more mental effort you apply to any given situation, the less will be the result.*

Initially, this may be difficult to accept. Your experience in the physical world indicates just the opposite: the more effort you apply, the *greater* the result. But in the mental domain, the more effort you apply, the *less* will be the result. You know this from your own experience – when you're trying to remember something that's 'on the tip of your tongue', when you're trying to solve a riddle, when you're trying to compose a speech, when you're trying to find the words to stop your lover walking out on you – the more mental effort you apply, the further away from the desired result you seem to be.

When you're calm, your mind is at its most potent. And no matter what your boss or professor may try to tell you, if you want to think well in your job or your studies . . . relax.

3. The Power of Substitution

Because the reasoning, analytical left sides of our brains dominate our everyday lives, and because we have been educated to believe in the might of the intellect, we tend to believe that all great improvements will be the product of willpower and conscious effort.

Your own experience will tell you this is not true. You have no conscious control over even the most basic levels of your thoughts. You cannot, for example, avoid thinking of a yellow Volkswagen with the number '6' on the side. Try it now. Force yourself not to think of a yellow Volkswagen with the number '6' on the side. You can't do it. It is impossible.

The only way of consciously changing a thought, or making a positive change to a habit or behaviour, is to substitute another. You can avoid thinking about yellow Volkswagens simply by thinking of something that appeals to you even more. Like what you're going to have for lunch, or the fabulous person you met in the supermarket last night, or how young you're going to feel next birthday.

You can avoid suffering from negative feelings – not by trying to suppress them, but by substituting positive ones. So instead of concentrating on the job you just missed out on, you concentrate on how much you're going to enjoy the next job you're going to find.

And you can overcome limiting behaviours by substituting enriching ones. So instead of concentrating on giving up smoking, you concentrate on becoming fitter and healthier; instead of concentrating on what you're forgoing (cigarettes), you concentrate on what you're gaining (new diet, new skin care regime, new exercise program, new wardrobe).

Substitution is immeasurably more powerful than willpower as an agent for change.

4. The Power of the Subconscious

In terms of controlling the way you think and feel, your subconscious is significantly more powerful than the total weight of your reason or willpower. Once the subconscious has taken on an idea, it immediately sets about turning it into reality. Your conscious mind cannot do that.

Your subconscious employs every resource you possess – all your mental powers, especially those you didn't know you had; all the observations you have ever made, including those you didn't know you were making; all the knowledge and information you have ever been exposed to that you have long since forgotten. In other words, your subconscious alone has the capacity to gather all your internal strengths – known and unknown – as well as all the forces of nature, to help create this (imagined) reality.

Whether it happens immediately or incrementally, it does take place. And it will do so for negative as well as positive reasons; it can make you depressed as well as happy; it can make you ill as well as heal you; it can make you fail as well as succeed.

> *To turn any idea into a reality, all you have to do is get your subconscious to take on the task.*

You consciously do this by abandoning willpower, then utilising one of the three influencers of the subconscious mind: emotion, repetition and imagination.

5. The Power of Emotion

We've spent more than 2500 years celebrating the majesty of the 'higher' mind: reason, intellect, writing and language skills. The 'lesser' mind – emotions, imagination and intuition – has been considered less important, preferably to be avoided altogether.

The fact is, if you want to effect positive change, knowledge means very little. Although the world of science and education wishes this were not the case, what you *feel* about an issue can be far more important than what you *know* about it.

> *Motivation comes from emotion, not knowledge.*

A whole lifetime of knowledge or information amounts to nothing on its own, if there is no feeling that accompanies it. (You probably won't even remember the information.) Yet, even the most trivial piece of knowledge can bring about extraordinary change when there is a strong emotion attached to it.

Just ask any politician or salesperson.

6. The Power of Imagination

A vivid imagination compels the whole body to obey it.
                                                      Aristotle

The most powerful way of influencing the subconscious and activating emotion is through the imagination. Indeed, as the picture-forming ability of the mind, the imagination is the main tool of the subconscious.

For example, I can give you 100 pages of data providing empirical evidence that there are no sharks in a murky lagoon you're about to swim in. But I guarantee I can make your blood pressure rise with one simple shark-attack story. Or by playing eight bars of the theme music from *Jaws*.

When it comes to how you feel, what you know is no match for what you imagine.

(And, to effect positive change, what you feel is infinitely more important than what you know.)

This is the way it should be!

Knowledge is based 100 percent on the past. It is never based on NOW, and it is not based on anything from the future. Imagination is based 100 percent on NOW or the future.

7. The Power of Repetition

The single most influential force that controls your attitudes, beliefs, capabilities and emotions is repetition – the words you silently use, over and over again, in your internal dialogue with yourself.

For this reason, one of the most powerful devices used in education, psychology and self-help is repetition. In its most well-known form, repetition is a key childhood learning method. 'Two times three is six. Two times three is six. Two times three is six. Two times three is six.'

Later in life, repetition again becomes a key learning method. This time we call it 'practice'. You practise your golf swing over and over and over again – until the action becomes so engrained in your consciousness that you never have to think about it. Once an action has become unconscious, you have the ability to perform it at a more refined level than if you were trying to do it consciously. Then, if you do think about it while you are performing it, the very act of thinking will limit its effectiveness. This applies to all performances in life – driving, singing, working, writing, golfing – the more engrained it becomes and the less you consciously think about it, the more effective it becomes. You know this from your own experience: practice leads to better performance.

(This process of engraining has a real physical dimension. Repetition establishes a fixed neural pathway in the brain, which dictates a mental activity and thus becomes a habit. See page 63 for more on how this works.)

Repetition is also effective in instigating change in other areas of life.

When you repeat a phrase to yourself – over and over – it becomes engrained in your subconscious and begins to direct your thinking and actions according to the words you use. This is known as self-talk, internal dialogue, or affirmation.

Affirmation works just as powerfully in the negative as in the positive. 'I'll never master this program.' 'I hate ironing.' 'Work is a pain.' These are sure ways of ensuring you'll never master the program, that you'll always hate ironing, and that work will always be a pain. Fortunately, though, the converse applies. 'This program is getting easier and easier to use.' 'I'm a great ironer.' 'I'm so fortunate to have work that is fulfilling.' These are sure ways of changing your thinking to the positive.

Intellectually orientated people usually baulk at the claim that affirmation is a powerful psychological tool. They often dismiss it as pop-psychological wishful thinking.

They are wrong. Affirmation works in exactly the same way as practice, mental rehearsal, repeated listening or viewing of instructive tapes, or repeated instructions from someone close to you. You won't need to be convinced of how easily a teacher or a parent can convince someone that they are brilliant or slow, handsome or plain, worthy or worthless, simply through the repeated use of words.

This is the power of repetition.

8. The Power of Focus

If party-goer A goes to a party and gets marooned in the bores' corner, their opinion of the party will be that it was boring. If party-goer B is immediately whisked into a room of extremely attractive, fascinating conversationalists, they will have an entirely different opinion.

If they are both reasonable people, party-goers A and B will be able to discuss their experiences and understand their differences in perspective. But, no matter how reasonable and understanding they are, just below the surface party-goer A will *know* it was a boring party, while party-goer B will *know* just the opposite.

Same party, different 'reality'. This is the power of focus.

If you focus on the pain in your ankle, it will grow worse; if you turn your focus to an intriguing movie on television, the pain will diminish.

Same pain, different 'reality'. This is the power of focus.

At any given time there are literally millions of things going on within you and around you. At any given moment, you can focus your attention (your awareness) on one, or at most, a few of these. What you are focusing on becomes your 'reality' at that time.

It makes no difference whether you intellectually agree with what you are focused on or not: it becomes your 'reality'. And we have already discovered just how subjective and flexible 'reality' really is.

Even the world of science is starting to acknowledge this.

'Nothing is real unless you focus on it.' (My simplified interpretation of quantum physics' Copenhagen Interpretation.)

'There are an infinite number of universes, each one corresponding to each person's view of it.' (My simplified interpretation of the Many Worlds Interpretation.)

For more on these, see www.calmcentre.com/reader; the password you need is 'reader'.

This is why businesspeople who consistently focus on negative economic reports in the media invariably do badly. This is why cyclists who focus on the inferior design of their bike frames consistently lose races. And why if you associate with mediocrity, you find it difficult to rise above it.

Fortunately, the converse also applies. If you focus on the good things in your life, you continually find good things taking place. If you focus on beauty, you see beauty everywhere. And if you associate with successful people, you somehow become successful.

Your focus becomes your reality.

This is one of the most important things to understand about mental change. If you want to change the reality you're focused on, simply focus on something better.

9. The Power of NOW

I confess there was a lot of argument over whether this particular power was a mental process or a philosophy. However, as it is the secret to becoming calm, utilising this calm state to effect other things, and enjoying life, we could hardly overlook it.

It is about the power of this very moment.

The ability to think discriminately about the future (imagination) is uniquely human; it plays an important role in creativity, competitiveness and even survival. However, it is not a recipe for happiness or fulfilment, and it is the playground of all worry and anxiety (both of which are future-based).

The ability to enjoy and get the most out of the moment is something we normally associate with animals or small children. How we envy their ability to be intrigued and fully occupied by a stick, an insect, or a piece of junk – with no thoughts on the future, what they have to do tomorrow, what's for dinner tonight, or whether they might get sunburnt.

You could be like that.

As you will know from experience, dividing your attention creates tension. What you may not be fully aware of yet is that concentrating your attention on only one thing is calming, fulfilling and efficient. When you dedicate yourself wholly to a task or pastime, immersing yourself in the detail and the execution, you create a similar state to that of meditation – your attention is centred, your mind is filled with one thing, extraneous thoughts cease, and you ease into the most profoundly relaxed and efficient state.

NOW has no time attribute. NOW allows no room for knowledge (the past), the imagination (the future), regret (the past) or anxiety (the future).

NOW cannot be thought about, analysed, or compared with any other event in your life – this can only happen retrospectively, after the moment has passed. NOW can only be experienced. If you experience it wholeheartedly, your life will be enriched. Moreover, you can usually experience it in any way you choose: you choose to be happy NOW, or calm NOW, or powerful NOW, or healthy NOW.

It's only when you look forwards or backwards in time that you impose limitations on yourself. 'I've been unhappy for three months; I must be unhappy now.' 'My illness is degenerative; I should be worrying now.' 'I've never enjoyed watermelon in the past; I can't be enjoying it now.' 'They won't give the position to someone untrained; I might as well forget about it now.' When you learn to live and to thrive in the moment, you are enjoying the peak experience of your life. Nothing compares. You are at your most powerful.

The Calm Centre's Nine Mental Powers have been the subject of many years' refinement. They are the keys to change, success and possibly even enlightenment. I suggest you make a note of these because, in essence, they are all you need to feel calm and in control of your life.

So far, you've discovered that:

- Being calm is a choice.

- It is easy to become calm – at will.

- From this calm state you can achieve extraordinary things.

- Calm and achievement are easier to gain when approached holistically.

- Your greatest power and your maximum potential come from your calm centre.

- You are totally centred when you exist in the moment – NOW.

- You possess Nine Mental Powers that can help you to enhance your life in ways you may never have believed possible.

5

CALM FROM THE CENTRE

Now you're going to discover a profoundly relaxed state known as Deep Calm.
From this state all sorts of things become possible . . .

Calm.

One way to discover the true nature of this word is to come with me to the remote heart of Australia. Even if it isn't the last place on earth, it can't be far from it. This is the centre of the Australian continent, the Outback. The driest permanently inhabited place on this planet. Indeed, it is so parched and unforgiving that even its deserts are encircled by deserts.

I spent my childhood not far from this place.

It is so flat here that a bend in the road becomes a landmark. At night, the canopy of stars is so alarmingly bright and close that you cannot help but see yourself as a part of the universe rather than an inhabitant of earth. This feeling is exacerbated by the inescapable aloneness. At night, car headlights can be seen approaching a full hour before they arrive.

Apart from a scattering of hardy bushfolk, and sometimes a few kangaroos around sunset, there are few signs of life here. The air is so still, and life so quiescent, that you can hear a fly approaching long before you can see it. From time to time, a distant crow might test its voice on the emptiness, but it will sound bored and non-communicative, as if just trying to affirm that life exists out there.

It's hot, too. When summer temperatures exceed 50°C, the locals might be moved to mutter, 'Bit warm today'. Visitors never say anything. What can you say when the air is so hot and dry that each intake of breath scorches all the way to the bottom of your lungs?

You will understand why few visitors come to the place where I spent my childhood. What incentive is there for tourists to drive 2000 kilometres from Sydney, travelling vast distances without encountering so much as a ripple in the landscape, only to arrive at a place where the only direction to go is *back*?

However, what makes the greatest impression on those who do make the effort is not the searing heat, the remoteness or the endless horizon.

It is the silence.

There is nothing in a city dweller's experience to prepare them for the immensity of central Australia's silence. It's not something subtle that creeps up on you after an hour or so – it is immediate and dynamic! It is like an infinite, auditory black hole. It is a silence that cannot be ignored. It distorts the eardrums, emphasises the heartbeat and effortlessly draws attention to itself. In many ways it is like the first time someone witnesses an earthquake, tidal wave or hurricane: a moment as exciting as it is humbling. Most visitors find it an awesome, possibly even frightening, experience.

But to those who are familiar with it, this silence is the essence of peace and tranquillity. Just listen, without expectation, and calm engulfs you.

This is the kind of calm I want to introduce you to. It's not a 'put your feet up and relax' state of calm, but a profound state of overwhelming peace. One that can only be found and experienced at your calm centre.

I call it Deep Calm.

From this state, many life improvements become possible – in health, longevity, spiritual fulfilment, success, peace of mind, contentedness, wisdom, relationships, happiness and prosperity. Everything.

Knowing how to access this state means that all of these opportunities open up to you. From this state you can choose to follow courses in life you might otherwise have believed were unavailable to you. You can choose to achieve things that assorted 'authorities' may have told you were impossible.

All from a state known as Deep Calm. That state exists, right now, at your calm centre.

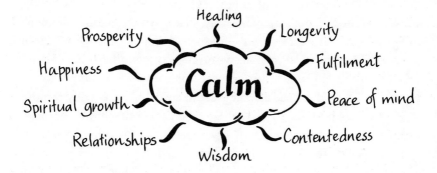

Some of what follows may seem rather simple to produce the kind of benefits you are expecting. The 'no pain, no gain' world that we belong to is suspicious of simple solutions. If they're so simple, how come everyone can't use them?

There are two answers to this. Firstly, everyone *can* use them. Secondly, while the starting point – Deep Calm – *may* be simple to achieve (and I emphasise *may*), the application of it can be as complex and as time-consuming as any other activity in life.

But, first, to this state of Deep Calm.

Over 5000 years in the design

Even after 20 years of research into meditation, neurofeedback, and the physiology of becoming calm, I base many of my techniques on traditional meditation.

There was a time when I taught just that. But, in the middle of a lecture one day, I was overcome with self-consciousness – it didn't seem right to be teaching the trappings of Eastern meditation when I had no cultural affinity with them.

It was then that I recalled my childhood. The town I used to live in had a population of about fifty. People spoke quietly (everyone speaks quietly and slowly in the Outback). You could walk from one end of this town to the other in about 4 minutes. Every student in the school could be seated in the one tiny classroom. No gas station, café, or cinema. One train passed through each week.

From as early as I can remember, my special place was on the out-skirts of that town. It was an old prickly acacia tree about 15 minutes' walk towards the horizon. The only shade worth talking about for miles. Try to picture this: you could stand under this tree and look around 270 degrees of horizon without seeing another tree, hill, or a feature on the landscape. Just endless horizon: red soil and blue sky, intersected by a dirt road heading off to somewhere equally remote.

There was nothing to do but sit there, sheltering from the fierce heat, listening to the sound of my breathing. No other sound, no distraction, just the sound of my slow breathing. After what seemed like years of this I had developed a new skill: the ability to become absolutely calm at will. Tranquil, absorbed by the moment, without need for distraction or stimulation, yet acutely aware of all that was going on around me. This was easy, because I felt I was at the epicentre of an infinite world. When this happened, I would find myself staring into an Aladdin's cave of opportunity and fantasy. (I recognise this state now as something akin to Deep Calm, where theta-open brainwaves are in the ascendancy and you are in touch with your subconscious.)

Although I wasn't aware of it at the time, there is an immense power that can be drawn from this state. It was only as I was gathering material for this book that I realised how immense that power could be. I recalled it being used for feats of healing. Of physical strength and endurance. Of business and artistic achievement. And, of course, for being able to remain calm. This is the power I call on to achieve my purpose in life – spreading calm.

However, I am digressing. A by-product of this experience was my recognition of the infinite nature of the world around me. By day, it was endless and awesome: undisturbed, yet constantly changing. By night this became even clearer. Even more silence, endlessness, wonder. Surrounded by all this, I was certain that where I stood was the centre of the universe.

Naturally, I am describing something that, at such an early age, was more sensed than understood. Or at least it was until one winter morning when I went exploring the town's dusty old railway stock-yards. Most of the year they were unused, and an Aboriginal stockman had set up camp there, unobserved by the rest of the town, probably waiting to pick up a job with a passing drover. I have no idea what his name was – or even if he told me – but, over the few weeks he was camped there, he changed my perception of the world.

The world I had known was a combination of tiny town and end-less nature. Then one poorly spoken, probably uneducated, stockman broadened the picture for me – not by telling me about cities, technology, wealth and cultural achievements, but by showing me the interconnectedness of people, the earth, the elements, the heavens and the spirits. In retrospect, the things he told me were most likely Aboriginal Dreamtime stories, but I still remember the details, because it was my introduction to the holistic nature of life.

I asked how it was that he knew about these matters – the earth, the heavens, the spirits, the past. I have never forgotten his reply:

'Listen.'

It has taken me more than 20 years to comprehend the subtle

meaning of that suggestion. Listen. When you accept the nature of silence, and think of it not as an absence of sound but as the presence of peace, you will be amazed by what you 'hear'. If you listen, *really* listen (in a state of Deep Calm), you will get an insight into the boundlessness of that which not only are you part of, but also are at the centre of!

This realisation was what motivated me to write my first book on meditation, *The Calm Technique*. That awareness did not prevent me from utilising the core strengths and understandings of traditional meditation practice. But it did mean I could omit much of the history, philosophy and mystical metaphors that were associated with it. You are not missing anything as a result of this; my methods have been well tested, consistently producing outstanding results, and some have even been adopted by the traditional meditation schools I emulated.

Why not use the traditional methods?

Even though meditation is relatively commonplace today, with millions of people participating or planning to participate, it still evokes a degree of confusion, frustration and possibly even suspicion. Why? Because it remains shrouded in the same mysticism and spiritual perplexity as it has for over a thousand years. I'm sure there were good reasons for this to have been the case – *once*. But, in this day and age, such mystification really gets in the way of effective communication. And severely limits the appeal of a practice that could do immense good in the wider community.

The polarising nature of the word

According to the ads, meditation can make a massive difference in your life. As a result, hundreds of thousands of people have paid – sometimes quite substantial sums – to learn how to meditate.

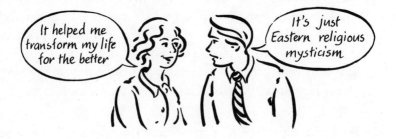

Yet people's reactions to meditation are still polarised. In many ways, the situation is not very different from when I brought out *The Calm Technique* in 1984.

The reason such polarisation exists, I believe, is a result of the way meditation has been promoted over the years. The mysticism that surrounds it has spawned as many detractors as devotees. As well, its association with Eastern spiritual schools, combined with the trappings of saris and saffron, has alarmed many of those allied to Western religions. I find it curious how meditation is almost exclusively associated with the East when it has also been part of Western religious tradition for thousands of years. Yet, for many, this Eastern flavour is part of its appeal. So the first degree of polarisation is philosophical. Or cultural. On the one hand you have those who are attracted to the spiritual exoticism offered by the older (Eastern) schools – and on the other, you have those who consider it a spiritual affectation.

As long as the word 'meditation' carries the associations that it does, this polarisation will continue.

In the techniques that follow, I will show you how to enjoy the physiological benefits that come with meditation – including, if you choose, the spiritual benefits – without asking you to subscribe to any particular philosophy or spiritual tradition.

We will do this through a normal, easily attainable state of mind known as Deep Calm.

Us vs Them

In the decades I have been researching and writing about meditation, one question arises more often than any other: 'Is X school of meditation better than Y school of meditation?'

I should confess that my responses tend to disappoint. Because, philosophy aside, my contention is that all meditation techniques are broadly similar. This is understandable since they have been influenced by similar traditions – Hindu, Buddhist, Taoist, Jewish, Islamic and Christian – particularly as they relate to monasticism. Although we don't hear much of them these days, the Gnostics also played a major role in the development of meditation practice, influencing many other religious schools (Roman, Persian/Islamic, Jewish, Christian). The techniques they employed were not unlike those found in the popular Buddhist and Hindu traditions: a search for divine inspiration brought about by an 'emptying of the mind'.

> *With the possible exception of hypnosis and biofeedback techniques, there have been few new developments in meditation practice for the past few hundred years.*

If you think the various schools of science and healing are partisan, they hardly bear comparison with the various schools of meditation – at least as far as their disciples are concerned. I suppose this is understandable. Often the way meditation is taught in the traditional schools is through a process of gradual enlightenment: this comes from the teacher, and the student is expected to follow the teaching without question, investing many years in rituals and activities of which they have little or no idea about the meaning. When the student seeks explanation, the response is often paradoxical or oblique – leading to further mystification. (The theory behind this is that when logic is exhausted, understanding begins.) The result? When someone devotes many years to a particular type of meditation and it serves them well, they can become a bit of a crusader.

In addition to this, psychology plays a part. Each individual habitually favours one sense or modality over another – visual, auditory, kinesthetic, intellectual – which means that any meditation technique favouring that particular modality will *seem* more profound to them. However, as far as I have been able to determine, one school of meditation is as good as another where psychological and physiological benefits of its practice are concerned. When it comes to the philosophical or spiritual benefits (assuming they offer these), that's another story, and one we'll consider later in the book.

While I understand the common argument that technique cannot be separated from philosophy in meditation, I reject it. The practice of meditation technique alone – without any philosophical or spiritual overlay – can be extraordinarily powerful and beneficial. Indeed, this is the experience of most Western meditators. (The greatest

number of Western meditators come from schools where the philosophy plays a very minor role, at least in the beginning.)

So, accepting that the technique of meditation is worthy of exploration, let's look at some of the practices that can bring about the
meditative state of mind – Deep Calm.

Deep Calm

Most types of meditation produce a specific mental state that I call
Deep Calm. The objective of the meditation process – while you are
involved in it – is to still your thoughts, and to unify your mind, body
and spirit for a brief period of total harmony.

The means of achieving this state of mind vary. But the state
itself remains fairly consistent – at least from a physiological point
of view. We can even measure it to a degree: galvanic skin response,
oxygen consumption, blood pressure, the balance of hormones and
neurochemicals, the levels of lactate in the bloodstream, and so on.
However the most revealing measurement comes from using an
EEG (electroencephalograph – see page 63) to plot brainwave patterns, the electrical impulses produced in the brain.

Using an EEG it is possible to determine the precise mental state
that accompanies the state of Deep Calm. (Not the mood or emotion; these can only ever be recorded subjectively, although some
emotional reactions do produce specific neurochemicals that can be
identified.) Generally, this unique state can be produced by an
experienced meditator and will involve elevated alpha waves, theta
waves and delta waves, and negligible beta waves (see page 68).

What this means is that the conscious (thinking) mind is quieted,
while the subconscious and the unconscious remain as active as they
always are – *but are more accessible to your understanding*. And this acces-
sibility is what provides the clarity of thought and inspiration that is
usually associated with being in a meditative state. While some consider this to be some sort of cosmic or divine intervention, you can
see how it is quite a natural and understandable human occurrence.

Deep Calm is more tranquil than the 'relaxed but wide awake'
state you are familiar with, but more aware than when you're asleep.
Moreover, Deep Calm is a unique state of mind brought about only

by meditation (and controlled emulation of this state using bio-feedback or various electronic devices).

What do you feel?

Let me describe the experience of Deep Calm.

For a start, you are relaxed in both mind and body. Your breathing and heart rate have slowed. Your body feels quite limp, almost floating. There is a sense of serenity and detachment unlike any waking state you have ever experienced. An overwhelming sense of peace and wellbeing. Thoughts have ceased altogether, yet you are totally aware of yourself and your presence in the world around you. Usually this is accompanied by a feeling of great certainty and security. From time to time you may experience moments of lucidity, wisdom, insight or illumination. Or sometimes this clarity is just a *sense* you carry with you the whole time, rather than something specific you are conscious of. The Deep Calm experience is pleasurable, satisfying and subtle. Sometimes the time will pass without your having noticed anything but at the completion of it, you will be feeling more alive, rested, aware, intuitive and contented.

If you were an experienced meditator, you would be familiar with this feeling. However, to be classified as an 'experienced meditator', you would have to have been practising on a daily basis for more than 20 years. Is it necessary to wait so long before being able to experience this?

Just wait and see.

While Deep Calm, or indeed any meditative state, is considered to be the product of many years of training and practice, it can be learned in a few minutes. Its unique psychological and physiological effects are surprisingly simple to reproduce: 'Instant Nirvana', as one London daily sneered, believing this was the ultimate put-down of the practice I am proposing. But it wasn't a put-down at all. You are capable of creating this Deep Calm state without the years of indoctrination and training. Most people can achieve it after just a few sessions. *All* people can get close to achieving it – that is, can reach the alpha stage of feeling calm and relaxed – in minutes.

How do I know? Firstly, because hundreds of thousands have

already learned how to do it. Secondly, because you are already familiar with the state of mind.

Your experience of Deep Calm

I will describe a few experiences that you will easily be able to relate to. You will associate these experiences with feeling relaxed and detached. Perhaps you would not have been particularly aware of any state of mind at the time; you were just . . . being. Probably you would not have associated them with waves of spiritual awareness – although, if you'd persisted over a period of time, you may very well have. The point I am trying to make here is that you have already experienced the state of Deep Calm, and it is both completely natural and easy to access.

Experience 1 You are enjoying the most beautiful sleep. Somewhere in the distance, someone is calling to you, telling you it is time for dinner or something of that nature. You can hear this voice, but you block it out, clinging to that wonderful sleeping experience like a child clings to its favourite toy. In that twilight world, you really appreciate the pure beauty of an innocent sleep . . .

Experience 2 You are lying face down on a table. You are naked, except for a towel draped across your legs. The room temperature is warm and comfortable, and lavender or some other essential oil is adding a pleasant, relaxing scent. Soft music is playing somewhere in the background, but you can't quite make it out.

Someone you feel very comfortable with is spreading warm almond oil into your back. They begin to massage your shoulders. Slowly. Firmly. Calmly. Their hands are warm.

The massage continues, stroke after relaxing stroke – for 10 minutes, 20 minutes, 30 minutes. You are aware of every stroke, yet there's not a thought in your head. No worries. No deadlines. No awareness of time . . .

Experience 3 You have a couple of hours to kill and are reading a new book. The story features a number of interesting, well-drawn characters and, as you read, you become more and more involved with one of them. You sense the things they sense. You feel the things they feel.

After a time, you glance down at your watch and realise that the sun has set, and a full hour has passed. You can't remember a thing that happened in that hour except that you were immersed in a story; you may not even recall the details of it, and yet you were oblivious to everything else . . .

Experience 4 The train has been moving through the countryside for over an hour. The picturesque scenery no longer registers. The clackety-clack of the carriage wheels can no longer be heard, but it continues. You are not sleeping: you are sitting upright and your eyes are open. But you are not awake either. Just sitting there. Relaxed. The repetitive rhythm of the wheels is easing you deeper and deeper into a state of relaxation. The sun is setting and you haven't noticed. You sense it, but you haven't consciously noticed it. You haven't noticed that your breathing rate has slowed, either, and that your eyes are unfocused. You are awake, but you haven't noticed a thing.

Some time later you become aware of the other people in the carriage once again and wonder what happened to the previous 10 or 30 minutes. All you know is that it was very relaxing and you didn't have a care in the world. As the scenery blurred by, the monotonous sound and the subtle swaying motion lulled you into another state . . .

In each of those instances, what you would have experienced was a trance-like state not unlike Deep Calm. Without any effort on your part, without any consciousness of particular techniques or mental attitudes, you would have achieved a state similar to that of meditation.

See how easy it is? See how effortless and pleasurable this relaxed state can be? In the first instance, you were on the fringes of sleep. In the second, you simply lay on a table while someone massaged you into a blissful, unthinking state. In the third instance, your imagination took over and you were 'lost in a book'. And in the fourth instance, you simply relaxed in your train seat, gazing out of the window, listening to the wheels, while you slipped deeper and deeper into a more tranquil state.

In essence, the procedure used to bring about a meditative state is as simple and uncomplicated as all of these examples. Despite all the efforts of meditation schools to turn this into a complex and mystical process, it is as simple as sitting on a train seat and watching the scenery go by. Or reading a fascinating book. Or reclining on a massage table and having someone rub your back.

Almost.

What I hope to show to you by the end of this chapter is that you can ease yourself into a Deep Calm state almost as easily. And, when you have made this technique part of your life, you will find it just as pleasurable.

The way to do this is to occupy your attention with just one thing – a word, a sound, an image, a thought, an action – until your conscious mind comes to rest, thinking is suspended, and your conscious mind blends with your subconscious and unconscious. And even though we speak of your thoughts being stilled, and your conscious mind being at rest, this is the one time when your mind is wide open . . . open to all the wisdom and understanding that lies, untapped, within you. This state is known as Deep Calm. While you are enjoying it, you can objectively observe the processes of your mind and body, flowing along with them rather than trying to direct them in any way. It is a wonderful, pleasurable, satisfying state. And, for those who attain it often, it can be profoundly transcendental.

However, it is a state that you cannot consciously reproduce. Let me emphasise that: *it is a state that you cannot consciously reproduce* – not by using the awesome weight of your intellect, nor all your willpower. You just can't do it; it is impossible. However, by filling your attention with just one thing, or by being lulled into a trance-like state by a rhythmic sound or movement, you can achieve it without any intentional effort on your part.

The six approaches to calm

Every form of meditation I am familiar with (excluding drug-induced meditative states), whether traditional or non-traditional, uses one of the following approaches, either singly or in combination:

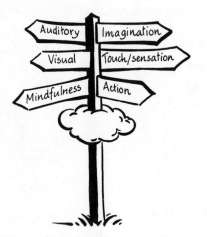

(i)   Auditory
(ii) Visual
(iii) Cerebral/mindfulness
(iv) Touch/sensation
(v)   Action
(vi) Imagination.

As far as technique is concerned, none is superior to the others. Each has its own advantages and disadvantages, often according to the type of person you are. For example, an outdoors, sport-orientated, active person may find more appeal in using action rather than imagination to attain Deep Calm. Similarly, an artistic, musically-orientated person may favour the auditory approach over touch/sensation. (Or maybe not.)

This brings us to one of the great fallacies of meditation practice. You often hear of someone changing from one meditation school to another in search of a teaching that is more in tune with their tastes, making a philosophical or spiritual decision on what 'feels right'. However, the perceived effectiveness of one school over another depends more on your psychological or physiological preferences than anything else. So if you've been meditating for 2 years and think it's not working for you, it may do to change your approach – though I can't think why you would persist this long if it wasn't doing anything for you, unless, of course, you were following an ascetic path. Fortunately, most traditional schools of meditation employ several approaches.

Auditory This is one of the most common techniques used in meditation. It ranges from music (choral, Gregorian chant, gospel singing, shamanistic drumming) to spoken words (Christian prayer, Indian mantras, Islamic dhikr) to *imagined* words. There are many old prayers which, when recited aloud, have a repetitive, drone-like quality that can induce a meditative state. Rosaries – specific prayers recited as beads are passed between the fingers – work in a similar fashion.

But probably the most widely known meditative technique uses a mantra. Used in Buddhism and Jainism, the mantra is generally considered to be Hindu in origin. It is a word or phrase, sometimes just a sound that is either spoken aloud, or imagined, over and over again.

Visual The visual approach plays a major role in most of the traditional meditation schools. Whether this is simply the iconography of meditation, such as the Hindu or Buddhist mandalas, staring at a candle flame, focusing on an object such as a lotus flower or a distant mountain, or watching whirling dancers, the result is the same: by occupying your attention with a single visual element, you gradually empty your mind of thought.

While we're on this topic, it is interesting to consider the design of the mandala. The mandala is a graphic representation, or plan, of

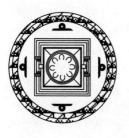

the universe – a focal point for its forces and energies that can be accessed through meditation. This is why it is often used as a subject of meditation.

Its general form is a square within a circle or concentric circles, and commonly featuring intricate formularised patterns. Sometimes, the Buddha or a deity is also featured.

The mandala pattern appears in other cultures as well – ancient Greek, Celtic, Native American, Australian Aboriginal, and Middle Eastern. Even Western psychologist Carl Jung dabbled with this image: according to Jung, drawing the mandala was an attempt by the conscious self to integrate unknown material from the unconscious.

Cerebral/mindfulness The cerebral approach tends to be more Western, whereas mindfulness is one of the foundations of the Buddhist meditation practice of Vipassana. Commonly referred to as insight meditation or mindfulness, Vipassana asks you to do nothing else but observe whatever manifests itself in the mind and body.

The intellectual approach I refer to is not some free-wheeling mental exercise. It is simply a way of consciously using your thoughts to stop yourself from thinking (don't you love the paradoxes that pervade in meditation?). The Zen koan is an example of this. Here, a meditator is required to 'solve' a paradoxical statement, such as 'the sound of one hand clapping'. Its purpose is to exhaust the will and intellect until the mind abandons analysis and begins to open up to a more intuitive perspective, giving way to the subconscious and unconscious. It works, but it can give you a headache.

Perhaps more accessible and user-friendly is the mindfulness approach. The intent here is not to avoid thoughts and observations, but to overwhelm yourself with them: you observe on a moment-to-moment basis everything that is going on about you – both externally and internally. Normally, you sit quietly and observe whatever comes to mind, or whatever feelings arise, dispassionately, in a detached manner, and as precisely as possible; you focus all of your attention on whatever is happening. While mindfulness is passive – in the sense that it does not seek to control or modify the thought or experience, merely to observe it – it is a very effective form of meditation. And it becomes more profound and more effective with experience.

Touch/sensation   Now we enter the world of the exotic. You've no doubt heard of the Tantric meditation practices (Vajrayana) which involve sex, or thoughts thereof, as a way of reconciling the spirit and the flesh. This is not part of mainstream meditation practice, but you can probably imagine how it might work – after all, love-making does induce a trance-like state in most people. As for making it a regular meditative practice . . . well, whatever turns you on.

Probably a more everyday touch-orientated approach to meditation is that which you find in reiki and shiatsu – deeply relaxing healing techniques where energy flows from the practitioner's hands to the recipient. Another area where touch plays a significant part in meditative practice is in the use of sacred objects such as the rosary and the prayer wheel.

Action   For many, physical action is the most accessible and convenient path to Deep Calm.

The traditional meditation schools that employ it range from Tai Chi to hatha yoga or any of the more athletic yoga styles, Zen walking meditation, and a whole range of dance-orientated practices – African, Caribbean, Brazilian, whirling dervishes, shamanism – in which fast, exciting percussive rhythms lead to a meditative state or even ecstasy.

Imagination   The final path to Deep Calm is the one I favour above all others – the imagination.

In many ways, it is used by all of the aforementioned approaches. Tai Chi calls on the imagination to describe its many movements – for example, 'grasp the swallow's egg'. In Hindu meditation, the chakras represent different parts of the body – the crown chakra, for example, represents our connection to our father, authority and God. Another popular way of using the imagination to produce meditative effects is through guided imagery – following either a spoken commentary or a simple hypnotic script.

However, the reason I personally favour the way of the imagination over the other methods is that it is very much 'today'. Its familiarity stems from the fact that it plays such a large part in our consciousness – not only is it the cornerstone of modern entertainment, it is also the most powerful tool of the subconscious.

Many paths   All the paths I have described come from classic meditation practices. Broadly speaking, each of them produces a state of mind similar to Deep Calm.

The appeal of one path over another depends to some extent on your psychological or physiological likes, but, without spending a lot of time in trial and error, how can you tell which approach is the right one for you?

By using your intuition.

In the pages that follow, I'll cover a range of different techniques. You can read through them, sample them, then choose the ones that appeal to you. That's all there is to it. Trust your instincts. Don't immediately go for the easiest (though instinctively most of us would do that), and don't cause yourself any anxiety over something that doesn't seem to be working for you.

Choose one from each of the following steps, and experiment with it. Once you have chosen a direction that you feel comfortable with, *stick with it*. Because perseverance multiplies the benefits over time. If, after you've done this for a while, you think you would be better served by studying with a traditional meditation school, then what you have taken from this book will serve you well.

So far, you've discovered that:

- **Being calm is a choice.**

- **It is easy to become calm – at will.**

- **From this calm state, you can achieve extraordinary things.**

- **You possess Nine Mental Powers that can help you to enhance your life in ways you may never have believed possible.**

- **Your greatest power and your maximum potential come from your calm centre.**

- **There are many paths to your calm centre and the experience of Deep Calm.**

6

A FEW STEPS,
MANY PATHS

This chapter contains many
calming techniques that can be
experimented with – individually –
over several weeks.
Take your time. Enjoy it . . .

Right now it is important to recognise that Deep Calm is not something strange and mystical, but a simple natural state that you have almost certainly experienced at other times in your life. A deeply relaxed state – nothing more.

All we are about to do here is to formularise it with specific techniques so you can reproduce this state whenever and wherever you choose to.

Many people would be aghast at the idea of falling into a somnolent state where they felt they had no control. They might squirm at the idea of being involved with something like hypnosis or strange rituals. But don't worry, this is about as far removed from what we are trying to achieve as I can imagine. You can choose to make Deep Calm as 'normal' and everyday as sitting on a beach listening to the sound of the waves. You're in control here. *You* get to decide how mundane or how profound Deep Calm will be for you.

As long as you are deeply relaxed and not thinking about anything in particular, you will be on the right path. And, if you decide you would like to become even more calm and relaxed, you will know how to do that at any time.

Now it's simply a matter of deciding which path you will feel most comfortable on. Fortunately, even this part of the process is simple and intuitive.

I have divided it into four steps. Each is easy to perform and should be enjoyable in its own right. And one follows another.

Step 1

Step 1 is essential. Ideally you will complete it in a beta-intense state, before even reading through the following steps.

β

Step 2

Step 2 offers you a range of options designed to work in their own right, and to form a bridge into Step 3. Experiment with these before settling on a few that work best for you. They will help you move into an alpha-relaxed state.

α

Step 3 presents another range of options. After you have experimented with them, choose one or two that you would feel comfortable making part of your daily routine. This state heightens your theta-open brainwave frequencies. Deep Calm follows. You can achieve most of what this book promises from this state.

θ

Step 4 is a permanent state of enhanced awareness. It is the refinement of, and the replacement for, all of the above. It comes after years of practice. It may be that you never actually get to this stage . . . If you don't, it should be seen as a choice, not a failure.

I continue to emphasise how simple and enjoyable these steps are meant to be. Even though the objective of each step is illustrated by a small graph of brainwave activity, this is not essential for your appreciation of the techniques involved. If you consider this too left-brain for your tastes at this particular stage, please disregard the technical information.

Step 1

You probably knew I was going to say this: the very first step on the path to Deep Calm is making the decision that you're going to become calm. Once you have done this, and particularly if you have done it with a degree of conviction, the path suddenly becomes a whole lot easier, clearer and more attractive.

Moreover, once you have thought about it and made the decision, you will already be some way down the path. And, right now, if we could monitor your brainwave patterns, we would see that a calm change had begun. It would probably be subtle, but it would already have begun.

I mentioned before how radio and television interviewers automatically begin to slow down and relax the moment the topic of calm is raised. The moment they begin to think about it. The moment they begin to talk about it. And they progressively become more relaxed as the topic unfolds. This is what will happen when you decide you're going to become calm. The more firm you are in your decision, the sooner you will begin to feel that warm sense of calm moving throughout your body. You will feel your thoughts slowing down, and your awareness increasing.

All it takes is a decision. The decision to become calm. Make the decision . . . now.

Are you starting to feel more relaxed?

Step 2

Now we can take that state of relaxation even further.

The objective of Step 2 is to modify your thinking processes – just a little – so you become even more relaxed. This should be restful and enjoyable in its own right.

When you have completed this step, you will be more receptive to even deeper states of relaxation, particularly Deep Calm. If you were to watch this process unfold on an EEG monitor, you would see a subtle shift from your normal waking brainwave state (predominantly beta-intense), to one that is more relaxed, untroubled and at ease (dominated by alpha-relaxed brainwaves). So, as you relax even further, the intensity of your beta-intense waves (thinking, concentrating) will be lowering, while the intensity of your alpha-relaxed waves (relaxing, open-minded) will be rising.

There is a range of simple activities that can bring this about. Some of them might seem a little odd, and I may be at a loss to fully explain why they work. But they *do* work – at least they do for most people. This last point is very important – 'for most people'. Norms are no longer applicable in this process. When we're talking about what goes on inside your mind, you're the expert; there are no standards you have to meet or norms you have to compare yourself with if you don't want to. It's important that you remember this.

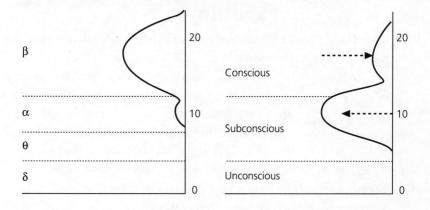

From Step 1 (normal waking) to Step 2 (relaxed)

Every person is unique. Every person works in ways that are special and powerful to them, and in ways that are mostly known only to them. In this context, no 'expert' in the world is more authoritative than you. What follows is simply what I have discovered works best for a range of people; only you can decide how it's going to work for you. But you always have the choice. And there will be many choices to follow. Providing it feels right for you, any of the following can be used in combination to enhance the effect.

Thought-stoppers

The best way to raise the levels of your alpha-relaxed brainwaves, and to help you feel more relaxed, is simply to stop thinking. When you stop thinking, there is an automatic and almost immediate change in how calm you feel.

The problem is that most people cannot just turn off their thoughts. 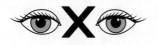 All the concentrated effort and willpower in the world cannot turn off a single thought. If it could, I wouldn't have had to write this book.

So, even though this is not a step you will have to take at this moment, it is something I had to point out early in the process.

Shutdown

The easiest and most obvious way of enhancing the alpha-relaxed state is simply to close your eyes.

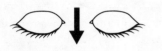

The act of doing this turns off much of your information processing – which is mostly visual – and has an immediate effect on your state of relaxation.

During neurofeedback, when people's brainwave activity is monitored, this one act produces the most consistent result. Simply close your eyes and you start to relax.

Try it now. Slowly lower your eyelids and take notice of how your body begins to relax – without your having to do another thing.

How did that feel?

Watch the Clouds

The next most reliable way of using the eyes to enhance this alpha-relaxed state is a step beyond closing your eyes.

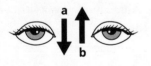

In this instance, *first lower your lids* (a), then allow your eyes to drift upwards (b) as if you were staring through your closed lids at a cloud just above the horizon.

When you are in a meditative state, your eyes drift up of their own accord. Similarly, in the moments before you fall asleep, your eyes tend to drift upwards. So consciously reproducing this action creates a similar effect. Why? I have no idea. Perhaps it's some psychological connection with sleep. All that's important, though, is that this simple action does work. For most people, it does create a restful state.

Try it for yourself. Close your eyes, then allow them to drift upwards. No effort, no straining, just taking note of the subtle feeling of relaxation that begins to overtake you.

Try it now.
How did that feel?

Widen your Vision

The final way of using your eyes to bring about, or enhance the alpha-relaxed state, is by changing your focus.

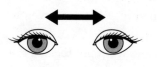

The task here is to widen your peripheral vision as much as possible, without moving your eyes. This process is known as deconvergence. Still looking ahead, allow your peripheral vision to broaden so that you can see more around you.

Why does this help ease you into the alpha-relaxed state?

I suspect it's a combination of two things: lessening the intensity of your focus and simulating the physiology of daydreaming. Try day-dreaming about something now. You'll find your peripheral vision automatically widens – though you wouldn't be aware of this unless I'd pointed it out.

Does that make you feel more relaxed?

Discover NOW

It will probably come as no surprise to you that people who have mastered the art of living in the moment, and who are comfortable with the passage of time, are much more relaxed about life.

Curiously, there is a simple way of achieving this without changing your thinking that much at all. All you have to do is remove your wristwatch (if you wear one), place it somewhere out of sight, then sit quietly, experiencing the moment.

Why do this? To put time into its proper perspective. The whole notion of time is artificial anyhow. The act of removing your watch is minor, I admit, but if you can look upon it as a signal to yourself that time is unimportant, that there are no time pressures unless you allow there to be, and that the greatest pleasure in life is simply being

– not waiting – you will find yourself beginning to move into an alpha-relaxed state in no time.

In this sense, the act of removing your wristwatch is metaphorical; it's a simple action you can take to remind yourself that you are master of, rather than a slave to, time.

Contact God

I have no idea how to explain this phenomenon, so I won't even try. Several years ago, researchers at the Calm Centre discovered that people could immediately put themselves into a deeply relaxed state by having sacred or holy thoughts – thoughts of, or communications with, their perception of God.

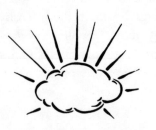 In more recent times this phenomenon has become so commonplace that researchers now refer to the 'God Spot' – a specific part of the brain that produces feelings of transcendence. When you access that part of the brain, you begin to relax into an alpha-relaxed state. Just by thinking of God.

However, we also discovered that other thoughts could produce a similar response. Thoughts of great love, for example, could bring about the same feelings of transcendence; so, too, could thoughts of magnificent scenery or works of art (for some people).

So the very things you think about have a direct impact on how relaxed you become.

Step Aside

Another interesting method of producing an alpha-relaxed state is to establish a more holistic view of your place in the universe (at this very moment).

This is not difficult. Turn your attention to the person who is reading this page. Now, turn your attention to the person who is sitting in your chair. When you can sense this, try to see yourself where you are now – but looking from outside of yourself. Try to imagine yourself sitting in the chair you're sitting in, reading this book.

When you feel comfortable with that, try to imagine the chair in relation to the rest of the room. And the rest of the room in relation to the entire building. And the building in relation to the street, the street in relation to the suburb, the suburb within the city, the city within the coastline, the coastline within the country . . . and so on, until you have a more holistic perspective.

What you will discover is that the wider your view, the more harmony, peace, silence and space prevails. All of these lead to calm. And an enhanced alpha-relaxed state. After you have tried this a few times, you can accomplish it very quickly, just by 'thinking holistic' – that is, as close to holistic as you can imagine.

The Floating Tongue

When I was researching *Instant Calm* several years ago, I became aware of the fact that tension in the jaw area (often accompanied by clenched teeth) was only present in the beta-intense state. Tense jaw muscles can lead to stiff back and shoulders, tension headaches, lower back pain, and overall feelings of tension.

My theory at the time was that if you could manage to relax your jaw muscles, then the relaxation would begin to spread through the rest of your body. Anecdotally, this proved to be correct; those who applied the following technique reported that they felt more relaxed. This was confirmed when we discovered that jaw-relaxing exercises promoted an increase in your alpha-relaxed brainwaves as well.

This is all about relaxing your tongue. Allow it to gently rest against the roof of your mouth, just behind your front teeth. The moment you do this, your jaw muscles will begin to relax. Another way is to imagine that your tongue is floating. One of my colleagues speculates that this discourages a condition known as sub-vocalisation, where you mentally articulate the thoughts and observations you are having, thereby locking yourself into a beta-intense state (which usually accompanies conversation).

Although simple, these exercises generally have an immediate effect on helping you to relax. Especially if you have a tendency to sub-vocalise and to carry tension in your jaw muscles.

The Uplift

If you're familiar with hatha or oki yoga techniques, or Tai Chi, you will be aware of how a simple posture or movement can help you feel more peaceful and relaxed. As it can take more than 2 years of practice to become proficient at these, my researchers were keen to discover whether a simplified version of these movements might also serve to produce a peaceful, alpha-relaxed state. A number were designed, and their effect on brainwave patterns was tested. Of these, four produced reasonably consistent results. They are included here for your consideration as Step 2 on your way to Deep Calm.

The first, the Uplift, requires very little physical effort and just a little imagination. Its purpose is to counteract the physiology of a tense person. You will be familiar with the look: slumped shoulders, dropped chin, stooped back, folded arms. You can release the tension simply by reversing those posture traits – by pulling back your shoulders, lifting your chin, straightening your back, loosening your arms.

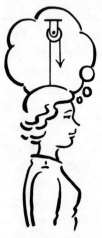

- To do this, simply imagine a single strand of thin, strong wire that's attached to an imaginary hook on the top of your head. Pass this imaginary wire through an imaginary pulley on the ceiling directly above.

- Then, imagine the wire being tightened . . . bit by bit . . . until your vertebrae start to straighten and you can feel your body beginning to lift.

- Continue, until you feel you are hovering a whisker above the floor.

- Your body will now be as straight as you can manage, yet it will feel lighter and more relaxed.

The more you can feel the wire lifting, the more relaxed your body will feel, and the more the alpha-relaxed frequencies will be present in your brain.

Lowering the Centre

In many martial arts, the initial posture is one designed to lower your centre of gravity. This has both defensive and offensive benefits, making you more difficult to throw and providing greater leverage for your attack. While it may seem an unattractive-looking pose, it is most effective in its application.

But it also has another effect. When martial artists lower themselves into this pose, with a hearty exhalation of breath, it immediately relaxes their body – centring them in a way that other exercises cannot.

You can use this same technique to enhance your alpha-relaxed response. (Do not attempt this one if you are very unfit.)

- Position your feet about a shoulder-width apart, with toes pointing ahead.

- Unlock your knees and allow your seat to lower (a).

- Keep your back straight (b).

- Allow your elbows to bend slightly so that you can feel a little space under your armpits. Let your hands dangle.

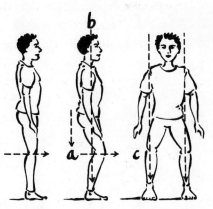

- *As you breathe out*, feel your body weight sinking towards your feet (c), pressing downwards until it anchors you to the floor.

You can enhance the effectiveness of this technique by combining it with the Uplift. Combined, they will help you to relax quickly – taking you a surprisingly long way along the path to Deep Calm.

The Feather-light Hand

Have you ever watched someone performing Tai Chi and felt calm and relaxed simply because you were watching?

While that may be an appealing prospect, the beauty of Tai Chi is not in the watching, but in the performing. For a start, it is almost impossible to feel tense while you're concentrating on the simple, connected series of exercises.

To master a complete Tai Chi routine takes time. And while you probably will derive benefits as you're learning, peak effectiveness comes after some years. Yet we have been teaching single Tai Chi exercises for some time now, with excellent calming results. So much so that the challenge was to see how much we could pare down one of these exercises while still deriving a calming benefit from it.

The exercise that follows is the result of that simple ambition. I should point out that, while this exercise was inspired by the graceful, balletic action of Tai Chi, it is not a Tai Chi exercise in itself, or at least it is not a complete one. It works as a calming step, though, because as well as slowing your movements down, it creates a physical link with your breathing rate – yet another way to relax.

Experiment with the following:

- If you are right-handed, do this exercise with your right hand initially. If you are left-handed, do it with your left hand first.

- With your forearm about waist level, palm downwards, slowly begin to lower your hand towards the vertical. As slowly as is humanly possible.

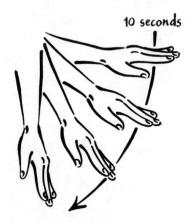

10 seconds

- While you do this, breathe out through your nostrils. Noisily, heartily. For 10 seconds or longer. *Concentrate on what this feels like.* Continue to focus on your hand until your fingers are pointing towards the ground.

- As you inhale, allow your hand to rise back to elbow height.

- When you can 'feel' the action that is required, and it is controlled by your breathing rather than by conscious effort, repeat the exercise with both hands at once.

The Art of Breath

Technically, this is not really a movement at all, but it probably has the most powerful calming action of all. In itself, it is very simple. Yet this one action is the forerunner to a process that most meditation schools acknowledge as central to becoming calm.

This is the process that I depend on more than any other for inducing and retaining a sense of calm in my life. Over and above all other techniques, I teach this to experienced meditators, novices and the chronically tense alike.

It involves breathing.

Breathing is an involuntary function of the body; it happens whether you're conscious or unconscious. It is unique in that it is the only involuntary activity that you have conscious control over.

By controlling the way you breathe, you can influence the way you think, your state of mind, health and wellbeing. You can use your breath to become calm, to heal, to overcome adversity, and to perform in ways you would not normally be able to. Most martial arts, meditation and yoga techniques are based around controlling the way you breathe. For thousands of years, these traditions have taught that by controlling your breath, you can influence your health, your strength, the way you think, and your state of mind.

To start with, you need to know how to take a deep breath. You probably know how to do this. Try taking a deep breath right now. Try it: the biggest, deepest breath you are capable of.

Did you try it?

If you did, chances are that you pulled in your chin, puffed out your chest, and lifted your shoulders as you filled your lungs. A big show of breath intake – lots of puff and noise – but it was not a very deep breath.

In the martial arts, and in Chi Kung and yoga, you learn that a deep breath happens in a very different way. A deep breath happens not up high in your chest, but deep down low in your abdomen. At the bottom of your lungs, through your diaphragm. The diaphragm is a sheet of muscle that separates the chest cavity from the abdominal cavity. The chest cavity houses the lungs and is surrounded by a protective rib cage with the diaphragm forming its floor. When you inhale correctly, the diaphragm contracts downwards, allowing the lungs ample room to expand. When you exhale, the abdominal muscles push the diaphragm up.

You probably knew that. But, chances are, you don't know how to breathe that way, and make your diaphragm function effectively, without considerable effort. Here's how to do it using your imagination.

To take a really deep breath, imagine the following:

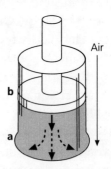

- Imagine that your lungs are a cylinder. Its sides are made from a solid material, and cannot expand or contract.

- The only flexible part of your imaginary lungs is a membrane – like a piece of balloon rubber – at the bottom (a).

- Imagine, when you take a breath, that the breath is being forced down into your lungs via a plunger (b).

- As the sides are fixed, and the air is being forced downwards, the only area that can expand is the flexible membrane at the bottom.

This is your diaphragm. It holds the key to breathing deeply. Learning to breathe deeply is only part of this exercise, but if you do it efficiently, you'll find your whole body beginning to relax.

One of the central understandings of martial arts is knowing how to breathe for peak efficiency. Interestingly, this type of breathing also produces the most restful, calm state.

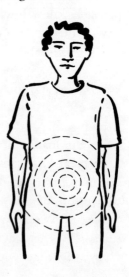

In a stressful situation, you will not have time to think about the technique I am about to reveal – you need to be able to do it intuitively. That is why it's important that you develop a *feeling* for how this works, and practise it a few times, before the need for it arises.

The essence of this technique is not so much an action as a mental approach. In other words, it all takes place in your imagination.

To begin with, the focus of your breathing

is right down low beneath your navel. This is where you imagine the breath forming. (The fact that you *know* it comes in through your mouth than moves downwards is irrelevant; we're talking about a feeling here.)

Once the breath has formed at the base of the lungs (diaphragm extended), imagine your lungs filling *upwards*.

Try it for yourself a few times and you'll discover that it makes all the difference when you're preparing to become calm.

(All this may seem a bit of a contradiction if you've studied some of the Indian techniques that encourage a light breath – 'so light as not to disturb the flame of a candle'. You'll find that my Chinese-derived method results in a similar lightness of breathing once you've reached Deep Calm, but makes it easier for you to achieve that state. In addition, some meditation techniques encourage light, rapid breathing. Although this does work for some, I am not a fan of it.)

Just Pretend

One of the fastest ways to become calm and relaxed is to have your subconscious take responsibility for the task.

As it is your subconscious rather than your conscious mind that encourages you to feel stressed and under pressure, it is appropriate that it should be the subconscious which is the most effective in reversing the situation. (See the Power of the Subconscious on page 100.)

Many of the calming techniques mentioned in this book depend on the subconscious for their effectiveness. In terms of controlling the way you feel, your subconscious is significantly more powerful than your conscious mind, and immeasurably more powerful than the total weight of your reason or willpower.

Unfortunately you can't get it to perform simply by instructing it to do so. The subconscious cannot be bullied – not by reasoning, logic, willpower, common sense or any other mechanism – into behaving the way you want it to. It must be *charmed* into doing what you want. In many ways, your subconscious behaves like an innocent – like a child. It functions best when it is entertained and allowed to play games.

This is why one of the most powerful ways to recruit your

subconscious into performance is to use one of childhood's favourite activities: pretending. Pretence is an immediate shortcut to influencing the subconscious, which is a shortcut to altering emotions or behaviour. By helping to create a new (imagined) reality this way, you can create new attitudes, habits and behaviours simply by acting as if they were already present.

You've seen the timid child who pretends to be bold fool himself into believing he is bold. You've seen the indolent worker who pretends to be ill really become ill. Now you can become the calm, tranquil, powerful person you've always wanted to be . . . just by pretending.

This is how it works:

- Imagine yourself as calm, relaxed and at peace.

- Tell yourself you have all the time in the world.

- In your imagination, note your slow breathing, unhurried speech, relaxed gestures, the hint of a smile.

- Now, start pretending you are exactly like the person in your imagination. Act as if you really were that person. Be as lavish as you like in this pretence – no-one will notice, only your subconscious.

- Remember it's important to speak as if you really were feeling the way you're pretending to feel. Use the words that relate to that kind of feeling. This helps make the change feel spontaneous and natural.

- If you want to take this further, imagine acting this way in a variety of different situations. Imagine yourself at work, at play, in social situations. How does it *feel* to be calm and relaxed in those situations?

- Next, pretend that others see you as the calm, relaxed person you're pretending to be.

Different steps to different tunes

This section has revealed just some of the many ways you can change your state from intense to relaxed – in a scientifically measurable way – simply by adopting certain attitudes, postures or actions.

There are many more. Here is a range of actions you can take to elevate the alpha-relaxed frequencies in your brain to help you become relaxed, while still being alert:

Smile It is interesting how the simple act of turning up the corners of the mouth into a smile can stimulate the pleasure centres of the brain and help you to relax.

One of the reasons this occurs is that smiling relaxes most of your facial muscles – the place where tension often concentrates. The other reason is probably because you've been training yourself since childhood to associate smiling with pleasure and feeling good. So, simply by affecting a smile you bring back those associations. (There are many studies that show how physiology affects mood. For example, sitting upright and smiling – even when you don't feel like doing so – helps to relieve feelings of depression.)

Essential oils You would think that, considering the level of information that exists on the subject of essential oils, no-one would ever need to encourage their use again.

Yet how many tense people do you know who overlook this powerful relaxation therapy? Essential oils do more than help you to feel good – some of them have a direct physiological effect, stimulating the production of neurochemicals that relax and uplift your mood.

You will discover that oils such as lavender, ylang ylang, rose, orange blossom and chamomile have a calming effect. Other oils to consider are cedarwood, lemongrass, sandalwood, geranium, bergamot, neroli, basil and patchouli. You don't have to be an aromatherapist to determine the most useful oils or blends: trust your instincts and your sense of smell. (This is a holistic approach to deciding what works best for you.) Use a few drops in an oil burner, or on a handkerchief, or in your bath water. And relax.

Incense Burning incense works in a similar way to essential oils. For most people, it creates a genuinely relaxing ambience. Considering that it has been used in meditative rituals for so many centuries, this should not be surprising.

Music As I mentioned before, music is an area of relaxation that I find particularly appealing – because it has the power to combine therapy and beauty.

You know from experience how powerful an effect music can have on your mood. But its influence is more profound than that: listening to music can produce real physiological changes in a person – altering the heart beat, breathing rhythm, blood pressure, hormone levels, brainwave activity, even the immune response.

There is a wealth of music – ranging from classical music to some of the more skilfully composed ambient music – that can help ease you into Step 2 on your way to Deep Calm. (For more information see www.calmcentre.com/reader, using the password 'reader'.)

Love As strange as it may appear, you can create deeply relaxed states simply by the thoughts that you have.

Those who have the wherewithal to have deep and loving thoughts about someone else will usually find themselves easing into an alpha-relaxed state very quickly. This same principle applies when people have thoughts of great reverence or transcendence.

Touch This may not always be the most practical exercise for you to attend to on an ongoing basis, but a gentle touch from another person works wonders in relaxing you.

The most effective way of achieving this is through intimacy with someone close to you. Another way is through massage or reflexology, both of which have the ability to take you straight through to Deep Calm without any effort on your part.

Visiting the centre

All of the techniques we will discuss in this book are designed to help you achieve a deeply 'centred' state – the same state that athletes, performers, therapists and martial artists seek to achieve before a decisive moment. This state is both relaxing and powerful.

When you can go to your centre at will, you have the means of establishing balance and harmony in your life. Meditators know that the most serene and satisfying place to visit during meditation is the centre. Or, more accurately, somewhere they *perceive* to be the centre.

It is not important that you can pinpoint this place in any meaningful way. It's not important that it even has a place at all. All that's important is that you can sense some place within yourself that you feel centred and strong.

Here is one way to sense, then go to, your calm centre:

- Sit comfortably, or stand, and pause for a few moments until you become aware of your whole body.

- Try to sense all parts of your body at once. Your limbs, your intestines, your heart.

- When you have even the slightest hint of this sensation, try to imagine your entire mass beginning to concentrate somewhere inside you. This may be in your head, or your heart, or your stomach, or at your feet – just move through these areas until one of them feels right. It can then be your centre.

- Now imagine all your thoughts, energies and strengths concentrating in that one point.

- That's all it takes for most people to feel centred, and to begin to relax.

The important thing to remember about the above techniques is that they're meant to be relaxed and comfortable. Enjoy them. Use them in combination. Lower your Centre as you use the Art of Breath. Widen your Vision and use the Floating Tongue, as you perform the Uplift. Enjoy yourself, treat them as an indulgence rather than a chore, and you will be in the right frame of mind to go on to Step 3.

Step 3

While Step 2 does serve a purpose in its own right – a range of calming techniques to enjoy and use to help you relax and overcome life's pressures – it has been designed as a warm-up stage, or as the bridge to Step 3.

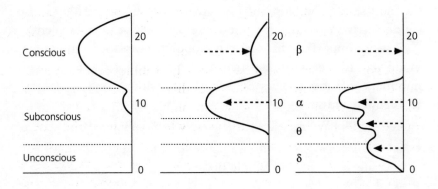

From Step 1 (normal waking) . . . to Step 2 (relaxed) . . . to Step 3 (Deep Calm)

When you follow the techniques featured in Step 3, you should find yourself on a simple, relaxing journey to Deep Calm.

Deep Calm, you will recall, is a state where you are more tranquil than 'relaxed but wide awake', yet more aware than when you're asleep.

As you can see in the graphs above, the stages in this process are:

- Step 1: a gradual diminution of beta-intense frequencies

- Step 2: a marked increase in alpha-relaxed frequencies

- Step 3: an increase in theta-open and delta-zzz frequencies.

Wild animals and meditation

Years ago, I heard this beautiful description of the mind's restlessness from a martial arts master. He compared the mind's random thoughts with untamed animals – they come and go as they please, regardless of what you ask or require of them.

The process of entering into Step 2 is akin to taking these untamed animals and tethering them to a central place. So, even though they still pull and strain and twitch about, there is an element of order to their actions. Step 3 is when you can direct these tethered animals to lie down, and rest quietly. So you no longer notice them.

The transition from Step 2 to Step 3 is sometimes accompanied by restlessness. You may develop an itch, or a flurry of thoughts, or a twitch, or impatience, or any number of distractions as you change states. For most, this is so subtle that it goes unnoticed. However if you do experience it, please remember this means nothing more than that you are moving from one state to another. And if you do experience it, you have a choice: either stay where you are in this state of semi-restlessness, or continue the journey on to Step 3.

Before we go any further, I want to refer you back to page 119, to the section, 'Your experience of Deep Calm', so that you can re-acquaint yourself with the sensation of being in that state.

Please pause for a moment – now – and refer back to that page. How do you feel?

Now it is time to move on to one of the most rewarding parts of this book – Step 3, a range of exercises that segue into Deep Calm.

In terms of psychology and physiology, Deep Calm is an identical state to that of meditation. You can choose to think of it as meditation if you wish, or you can think of it as Deep Calm if that *feels* more comfortable for you.

Either way, it is a thoroughly enjoyable place to be . . .
mentally and physically at ease . . .
your breathing rate slow and relaxed . . .
body quite limp, almost weightless . . .
a sense of serenity and detachment . . .
an overwhelming sense of peace and wellbeing . . .
no thoughts, yet totally aware of yourself and your world . . .
a great feeling of certainty and security . . .
clarity.

At the completion of 20 minutes of this, you will be feeling on top of the world: alive, rested, aware, intuitive and contented. Just as importantly, this state will provide you with the capacity to perform things you might never have thought possible.

Step 3 again presents you with a range of options: choose a few of them according to what feels right. Experiment with them. Then, choose one or two that you could comfortably make part of your daily routine. When Deep Calm becomes part of your routine, all things are possible.

Extending time

There will be a giant chasm between those who will make the following techniques work for them and those who won't. This will not be a question of belief or understanding; it will be a question of commitment. Most in this latter group will say, 'I don't have the time'.

This is not unusual. That belief has moved way beyond cliché and has almost reached epidemic status – the vision of cities swarming with people who don't have enough time to do the things they need to do would be almost comical, if it weren't so serious.

This concept of time running out is nothing more than a perception. There is ample time available for whatever we have to do. Eons and light years of it. I'm going to share with you two pieces of advice that could help you discover you have all the time in the world.

The first is a calculation. The second is an affirmation.

The calculation How much time a day do you devote to gossip, watching television and reading the newspaper? Be honest now: does it amount to 1 or 2 hours a day?

Give me 1 hour.

If you devote just 1 hour a day to the enrichment of your life, you'll find you have 365 hours a year. That is 9 working weeks.

Just imagine if someone handed you 9 working weeks to work on anything at all that you considered important. Imagine what you could achieve in 9 working weeks. No time pressure. No thought of time running out.

Why, you'd feel you had all the time in the world.

The affirmation Affirmation is a technique used by hypnotherapists, psychotherapists, promoters of self-improvement courses, and people who want to change their own attitudes or behaviours. When you use it yourself, this is known as self-instruction or auto-suggestion. It is also key to one of the Calm Centre's Nine Mental Powers: the Power of Repetition.

Affirmations are sets of words that derive their power from repetition. As these words are repeated over and over, they begin to influence the subconscious and become self-fulfilling, with the meaning of the words or sentiments you choose determining the results you achieve. Affirmation can be a powerful tool for change.

Generally, I am not a great advocate of it. I did a survey of people who had read about, or had been taught how to use, affirmation techniques and found that hardly anyone used them to any degree. So, while we acknowledge that they have power, and we know they can influence the subconscious, they have failed in the motivation department. This is the reason I am reluctant to recommend them.

Except in this one instance.

There is one affirmation that I use myself, and encourage all people to adopt and apply several times a day. When you read it, you will see how you could work it in to your inner dialogue so that it becomes part of your consciousness.

The affirmation is: *I have all the time in the world.*

When you first read this, you will say to yourself that it can't possibly be true. But once you try it a few times you will be convinced. Even if you are chronically unpunctual and a procrastinator, there is every likelihood that you feel time pressures just as much as everyone else. If so, repeat this phrase to yourself whenever the opportunity arises: *I have all the time in the world.*

You will note that most of the Step 3 techniques that follow use this thought at the outset. *I have all the time in the world.*

The different approaches to Deep Calm

As in meditation, there are six general approaches that will help you reach Deep Calm: Auditory, Action, Touch/sensation, Mindfulness, Visual and Imagination. As with Step 2, they can be used singly or in combination.

The object of all of them is to still the mind and clear it of conscious thought. Why? Because when you stop thinking, the beta-intense activity of your brain automatically decreases, and the alpha-relaxed waves increase. Then, you can relax and simply 'be'.

The process of stilling your thoughts is a straightforward psychological process whereby you fill the mind with one basic element (such as a word or image or action) so there is no room for any other conscious activity in your mind. This is exactly how meditation works. This is how prayer and religious contemplation work. This is how Deep Calm works.

To understand why it works this way, we need to consider exactly what thought is. The nature of thought is to be restless and always on the move. Like an electrical impulse running down a wire, it depends on movement for its existence, always heading from one place to another. Moreover, you cannot stop it or slow it down simply by applying conscious effort.

The third of the Calm Centre's Nine Mental Powers, the Power of Substitution, tells us that the only way of consciously changing a thought is to substitute another. In the case of Deep Calm, where the objective is to eliminate thought altogether, the only way of consciously doing this is to substitute something else that can occupy the mind. This could be an image, a fantasy, a feeling, a repetitive action, or even a *sequence* of thoughts so that the direction of your thinking is focused and limited. Or it could be a single word or phrase.

When you centre your mind or attention on only one thing, thought ceases. (Remember that thought depends on moving from one thing to another for its existence. When there is no movement, there is no thought.) So filling your mind with only one thing is tantamount to having nothing on your mind at all. The restless nature of thinking is slowed, and your mind is free from unsolicited thoughts. Only consciousness remains. This is the most peaceful and most creative state you can experience.

Each of the techniques that follow will help you achieve this state. The challenge is to find the one, or ones, that most appeal to you – and your best ally in determining this is *intuition*. What *seems* right to you? As you read through these techniques, or experiment with them, which ones *feel* right?

If you want to see which one you should try first, spend 30 seconds performing the following exercise.

- Imagine a helicopter lifting off the ground just in front of you.

- It's a midsummer's day. You are just out of reach of the helicopter's rotor blades, which are beating furiously.

- The helicopter begins to lift off the ground.

- Before you read the next paragraph, close your eyes and spend a few seconds imagining the situation you have just read about . . .

Have you done it?

For most people one sensation would dominate their experience of this imaginary situation. That sensation would (probably) have been along the lines of:

 (i)   they would have 'seen' the helicopter, the sun glinting on its glass, the green of the grass; or

 (ii) they would have 'felt' the wind from the rotors, the midsummer sun on their face, the grass under their feet; or

 (iii) they would have 'heard' the powerful engine and the spinning of the rotors over and above all else; or

 (iv) they would have 'thought' about what a strange way this is of determining which calming techniques they should try first.

Knowing which of your senses tends to dominate can make it easier to settle on the most comfortable techniques for you.

If you most related to (i), it may be better for you to explore the 'Visual' and 'Imagination' techniques first. If your experience was (ii), it may be better for you to explore techniques involving 'Action' and 'Touch/sensation'. If you most related to (iii), explore 'Auditory' first. And if your experience was closest to (iv), you might consider 'Mindfulness' first.

This is a crude barometer of your preferences, so please keep an open mind regarding the others. You never know, the one you end up feeling most comfortable with may be one you least suspect at the beginning.

Before you perform any of the following exercises, remember to use one or more of the techniques from Step 2 – this will lessen the time required for Step 3 to become effective.

A Word of Calm

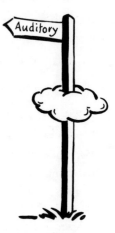

One of the most common techniques used in meditation is the spoken word – the repetition of a single word or phrase until you move out of your restless state into one of great peace and calm.

It can be any word you care to invent. A word chosen at random from the dictionary or phonebook. Any sound you fancy. If you can't think of a suitable one, use 'calm'; or, more restful and melodious still, 'calming'.

For the technique that follows, all that matters about the word you choose is its repetition. It is either spoken aloud, or imagined, over and over again. I suggest you speak it aloud for a minute or so, until you're used to hearing the word spoken in your own voice, then imagine it from there on.

If you have trouble coming to grips with this exercise, ponder the following metaphor: your mind is a roomful of shouting people. Among all that cacophony is a single voice you recognise. Listen to that one voice – your voice, your mantra.

That's all there is to it. In your mind, hear yourself saying this word over and over again. When your attention strays – which it will – simply coax it back to the word. This is not meant to be a strain; calmly redirect your attention back to that word when you become aware that it has strayed.

- Sit somewhere quiet where you won't be disturbed, preferably on a comfortable, straight-backed chair.

- Close your eyes and listen to the sound of your breathing.

- Tell yourself, with as much conviction as you can manage, that you have all the time in the world.

- When you feel relaxed, hear the word you have chosen coming from somewhere inside your head – as if you were speaking it yourself. If the word is 'calm', imagine you can hear yourself speaking it.

- As you breathe in, listen for the word 'calm'; as you breathe out, hear the word 'calm'. That is all you have to do.

- When your attention wanders, calmly redirect it to the word – when this feels comfortable.

- Continue this for 20–30 minutes.

Please remember, this is meant to be relaxing. It is a pure experience of NOW, nothing more. It is not a competition, nor a test of concentration or willpower. It is simply an experience of NOW. Of simply being.

I have linked the sound of the word with the sound of your breathing. The only purpose of this is to help you establish a rhythm – which is unimportant in itself, but may remove one extra thought from the process. If you feel uncomfortable synchronising with the rhythm of your breathing, simply avoid it. Just listen to the sound of that imaginary word.

(For a more complete understanding of this technique, read my earlier book *The Calm Technique*.)

The Breath of Calm

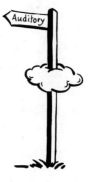

Although I have included this technique under 'Auditory', it could just as easily apply to 'Touch/ sensation' or 'Imagination'. Like many of the techniques in this section, it involves a number of senses.

The Breath of Calm is based on a yoga technique. In another sense, it is based on Tai Chi or Chi Kung; or perhaps you will recognise it as a Zen Breathing Meditation. In any event, you will be able to master this technique in just a few minutes. It involves three simple steps.

Breathe deeply One of the fastest ways to relax the body and start focusing the mind is to breathe deeply. The way to do this is to imagine that the sides of your lungs are fixed and that the only flexible part of them is at the very base – your diaphragm.

As you breathe in, the sides of your lungs do not move, but you can feel the flexible diaphragm expanding. If you place your hands on your hips when you take a deep breath, with your forefingers almost touching your navel, you should feel them beginning to lift as your lower stomach swells. This is a deep breath. This is the first step to Deep Calm.

Breathe slowly If you've ever compared the breathing patterns of a calm person with those of a stressed person, you'll notice a significant difference in their rate of breathing. The stressed person will breathe quickly, in short, shallow breaths. The calm person will breathe slowly. Depending on how relaxed they are, they might breathe around 5–10 times a minute.

So, once you've started breathing deeply, to become even more relaxed all you have to do is breathe more slowly. Not so that it becomes a strain or an effort – just to keep this concept of breathing slowly in the forefront of your mind. (You'll find your breathing rate will gradually slow down – without effort – when you think this way.)

Listen This last step is the one that turns a simple, 2-minute breathing exercise into a profoundly calming experience.

This element is so deceptively simple that you may mistake its simplicity for a lack of power. Yet this technique is among the more powerful I know. With minimal variation, it is all that is taught in some schools of meditation for the first couple of years.

All you have to do is listen. Listen to the sound of your breath as it comes and goes. Listen to the inflow of air through your nostrils. Listen to the sound of your warm breath as you breathe out through your mouth.

Here's how it works in practice:

- Sit somewhere quiet and restful where you will not be disturbed for 20–30 minutes.

- Tell yourself you have all the time in the world.

- *Listen* as you breathe deeply. In through your nostrils, right down low until your lower abdomen swells. Out through your mouth – noisily.

- *Listen* as you breathe slowly. In through your nostrils, lower abdomen swelling. Out through your mouth – noisily.

- *Listen* as you breathe in deeply, forcing the oxygen into the extremities of your body – your hands, feet and skull. Feel it coursing through your bloodstream to these parts.

- *Listen* as you breathe slowly, feeling the tension flood out of your body into your chair or the floor.

- *Listen* as you breathe deeply, the air forcing strength and energy into every part of your body.

- *Listen* as you breathe slowly, feeling your muscles relax as the tension flows out.

The Breath of Calm is so simple, yet so powerful. In essence, it requires little more effort than: breathe deeply; breathe slowly; listen. It's as easy as that.

There is another benefit to using the Breath of Calm. You can use it in the most unlikely environments. Simply by listening to the sound of your breathing 'inside' your head, it will help you to relax in the noisiest conditions. If you listen for it, you will hear it. Clearly.

Try this for yourself now. Wherever you are, whatever you're doing, take a deep breath, and listen to the sound of your breath as it comes and goes. And relax.

Enhancing the Breath of Calm

One of the postures used in Buddhist meditation can help you to feel even more relaxed. Lightly lay the back of the right hand in the palm of the left and let both hands rest on your lap. Then continue with the Breath of Calm.

Calm Sounds

Music is a powerful way of using sound to ease yourself into deeper and deeper levels of relaxation. It can work, without any effort on your part, at the same time as it gives you pleasure.

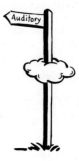

There are two ways it can do this. The first is through the emotions: simply listening to music can alter your mood. The second is more physiological in the way it works and is, therefore, more predictable in its effectiveness.

Certain sound frequencies can influence the frequencies of your brainwave activity to induce relaxation, arousal, concentration or any number of other states. They do this through a process known as entrainment.

Entrainment is fairly straightforward in principle: if you take an A Major tuning fork and tap it, any other A Major tuning fork nearby will resonate in harmony. The electromagnetic waves in the human brain can be influenced in a similar way. If the brain is exposed to specific frequencies – mainly through your hearing – it can be entrained. Thus, if the frequency happens to correspond with alpha-relaxed frequencies, your brainwave activity can be coaxed to adopt that state. In this way, the tones and rhythms (frequencies) of a musical composition can not only help a listener to relax, but can encourage much deeper states.

There are a variety of ways in which Deep Calm can be accomplished by using sound directly, or by using it in conjunction with other techniques.

Music Many of us have experienced transcendental or even rapturous states while listening to the works of great composers, gospel singing, Gregorian chants, sacred and other types of music. For most of us, though, the impact of this is sporadic at best.

There is another, more dependable, kind of calming music. This is not the wishy-washy 'ambient' stuff, which normally does not help you progress beyond the Step 2 relaxation levels. The frequencies required to produce a state such as Deep Calm are extremely low in range – from 1 to 12 Hz (cycles). This is way beneath the range of normal human hearing.

Because of this, conventional musical composition cannot reproduce the required entrainment effect. However, by *combining* the frequencies of two different tones, a third frequency is produced (although it is not perceived as a tone). This is known as a 'binaural beating' and can entrain the brain in exactly the same way as any directly produced note. Very few composers have the artistic and technical abilities required to produce music of this nature that succeeds on creative as well as technical levels.

There are also non-technical ways of using music to facilitate Deep Calm states. For example, there are certain musical instruments which, in the hands of well-trained intuitive musicians, can produce profound calming effects. The Japanese shakuhachi, or Zen flute, and the didgeridoo can work in this fashion, as can the chants of Tibetan Buddhist monks. Similarly, shamanistic drummers often use specific rhythms (principally 4.5 beats per second) to induce trances in their listeners, and use different rhythms to produce different effects.

From year to year, we come across musicians who succeed in this area. We endeavour to maintain a representative selection of these on the Calm Centre web site, which you can explore at any time: www.calmcentre.com/reader, entering the password 'reader'.

Sound As the frequencies required to produce Deep Calm are outside the normal hearing spectrum, it is always a challenge to find creative ways of reproducing them.

One way the entrainment effect can be produced is by using headphones. If, for example, you play a 300 Hz tone in the left ear, and a 310 Hz tone in the right, the effect *inside your head, at the brainstem* is the difference between these tones – in this instance, 10 Hz (310 - 300 = 10). These are known as binaural beats, and represent a clever way of producing sounds, or at least the *perception* of sounds, that are outside the normal hearing spectrum.

But this is far from anything you'd call music – and is not usually an enjoyable listening experience. However, as a means of inducing a calm state, it can be very effective.

Once again, if this area of sound entrainment interests you, you will find a representation of it at www.calmcentre.com/reader.

Light and sound Another non-musical method of producing Deep Calm is through the use of specific rhythm patterns. An electronic machine is used to produce a specific number of beats per second – for example, six beats per second to produce a six-cycle effect – which can entrain the brain in the same way that a tonal frequency would.

To make this effect even more pronounced, these rhythm-producing machines usually have a visual component as well – operating via special glasses which flash tiny light-emitting diodes at the same frequency. Known as sound and light machines, or mind machines (or variations thereon), there are many different makes available.

The states they can help you experience range from peak-performance through to sleep-inducing. Many find they can lead to Deep Calm faster than natural methods. With practice, though, you will find natural methods work every bit as quickly. At the Calm Centre, we have conducted experiments with several of these devices; check out www.calmcentre.com/reader for the most up-to-date information.

Dolphins and whales I had always thought the New Age fascination with dolphins and whales was the aquatic equivalent of an obsession with alien abduction. However, having met several scientists working in this field of research, I am convinced that one of the most elegant forms of brainwave entrainment occurs in the proximity of these animals.

In other words, when you swim with dolphins or whales, you find yourself easing into a synchronised state almost immediately. Dr Peter Beamish, a Newfoundland-based researcher in this area, believes that this is the result of communication efforts between dolphin and man (or vice versa). Since their perception of sound waves is thousands of times greater than our own, it is feasible for them to receive and initiate brainwave patterns from distances of a hundred metres or more.

Certainly the anecdotal evidence of divers in this situation leads me to believe that there are extraordinary possibilities inherent in this form of 'calm communication'.

The Calm Walk

Wouldn't it be ideal if you could combine your daily exercise program with the process of moving into Deep Calm?

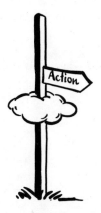

This is not only possible but is part of the attraction of this technique. I use it myself most days of the week.

The reason I am so enthusiastic about this particular technique is that it has a dual benefit – an exercise benefit, and a calming benefit.

The Calm Walk utilises an action that you intuitively use when stress becomes overwhelming – you start to walk, or to pace. Your unconscious mind knows that walking is one of nature's great antidotes to stress, a neat way of dealing with those chemicals your body produces in stressful situations.

In its most basic form, the Calm Walk is little more than going for a stroll or, if you prefer, a brisk walk. (Choose the pace that works best for you.) You don't have to close your eyes and you don't have to perform any attention-grabbing rituals. Yet you do become deeply relaxed, without having to invest any significant effort outside your normal walking action.

The steps are simple.

- Before you begin this, plan your walking course. It should take 30–45 minutes. (This is a little longer than most of the other Step 3 exercises, as it takes a few more minutes to start creating the effect you want.) Walk the course a few times before beginning the exercise, so that you are familiar with it.

- For obvious reasons, it is better *not* to do this beside dangerous cliffs, in unfamiliar territory or near busy traffic. A large park, the beach or countryside would be ideal.

- Firstly, tell yourself that you have all the time in the world.

- Widen your peripheral vision, as described on page 133.

- As you begin to walk, let your eyes rest about 2–4 paces in front of you, and just slightly to the right (for exact placement, see

'Where to rest your eyes' below). At the same time, ensure your peripheral vision remains wide.

Where to rest your eyes

Central to the effectiveness of this exercise is knowing the precise place to rest your eyes as you walk.

There is one place that will feel absolutely right to you. It will probably be 2–4 paces ahead, just slightly to the right. However if it is further ahead, or slightly to the left, that is a matter of personal choice.

To discover the ideal position, try to feel your foot *inside* your shoe as you walk. Be aware of this sensation. When you can sense it most distinctly, note where your eyes are resting. This is the ideal place for you to rest your eyes.

- While you are walking, listen to the sound of your breathing. Concentrate on the sound of your breath as it comes and goes. Keep concentrating on this sound. (If you're in a noisy environment, you may think this impossible, but you'll be surprised how easy it becomes after a few minutes – it's almost like listening to yourself breathe under water.)

- When your attention wanders, calmly bring it back to the sound of your breathing.

- An alternative to listening to your breathing is to mentally say to yourself 'left', as your left foot touches the ground, then 'right', as your right foot touches the ground. Or you can count each footstep up to eight, then over again. 'One, two, three, four, five, six, seven, eight; one . . .'

- Continue walking as evenly as possible while you listen to your breathing (or counting) for 30–45 minutes. Even though you will not be paying attention to this, you should be fully aware of all that's going on around you at this time, so you needn't worry about bumping into obstacles.

It may take you a few weeks to be able to reach the Deep Calm state as you walk, but it does happen. And once you have mastered it, the Calm Walk will become a favourite.

Even though the above technique uses walking to focus your attention, other forms of exercise can work just as efficiently. Swimming, jogging, rowing, Tai Chi – in fact any form of repetitive, unthinking exercise at all – can produce similar states. Whatever you feel most comfortable with is the right one for you.

Enhancement #1 – lowering or raising

Once you have become familiar with the Calm Walk, and you can do it without thinking about what it involves, it is time to enhance it.

You can do this by choosing one of the following:

- Before you begin walking, Lower your Centre, as described on page 137. It is not important that you maintain this posture, just that you keep in mind the centred feeling this posture encourages.

- Maintain this centred 'feeling' as you walk, pivoting from the hips, so that you feel your centre of gravity closer to the ground.

- Alternatively, before you begin walking, use the Uplift on page 136. Try to keep this *lifting* sensation in mind as you walk, so that it feels as if you are suspended just a small distance above the ground.

Some meditation teachers believe that trying to combine a calming exercise with a physical exercise is a compromise. Perhaps it is for some, but I find it most effective.

If you can make it work – and only experience will tell you if it does work well for you – it is a great way of incorporating the two activities into a busy lifestyle.

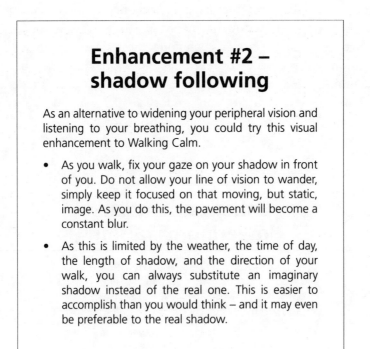

Enhancement #2 – shadow following

As an alternative to widening your peripheral vision and listening to your breathing, you could try this visual enhancement to Walking Calm.

- As you walk, fix your gaze on your shadow in front of you. Do not allow your line of vision to wander, simply keep it focused on that moving, but static, image. As you do this, the pavement will become a constant blur.

- As this is limited by the weather, the time of day, the length of shadow, and the direction of your walk, you can always substitute an imaginary shadow instead of the real one. This is easier to accomplish than you would think – and it may even be preferable to the real shadow.

Total Awareness

The intention of Total Awareness is simply to overwhelm your senses with all that is going on in the world around you – the sights, sounds, feelings and sensations. Then, by eliminating these one by one, to narrow your attention further and further, until your thoughts are stilled and you reach Deep Calm.

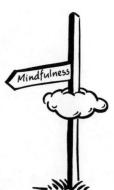

- Sit quietly in a dimly lit room. Loosen your clothes, make yourself comfortable, and just relax.

- Tell yourself you have all the time in the world.

- Imagine yourself at the very centre of your world (see 'Journey to the centre' on page 87). All you are seeking here is a sensation, an awareness of being in the centre. This will probably take a couple of minutes to accomplish.

- Focus on one bright spot in the room. Fix your attention on that highlight.

- Widen your peripheral vision until you can take in most of the room.

- Now, *without moving your eyes*, note six different things you can *see* in that room.

- Without allowing your eyes to stray from the highlight you are staring at, note six different sounds you can *hear*. (The birds in the trees, a car going past, the tick of the clock, your own breathing, etc.)

- Then, without allowing your eyes to stray from that highlight, note six different things you can *feel*. (The chair beneath you, your hands on your lap, the soles of your feet on the floor, etc.)

- Next time around, note only five of those things you can see. And hear. And feel. (All the while focusing on that same highlight.)

- Then note only four things.

- Then three. And two. And one.

Chances are you will lose yourself in a deeply relaxed state some time before you get to one. If, however, you are still consciously aware of your surroundings at that moment, simply repeat the exercise.

Like the other techniques in Step 3, Total Awareness has no purpose of its own – other than to clear the mind of thought. The object is to fill the mind with observations until you stop thinking about the observations. Then your mind becomes still.

Strokes of Calm

Here is a foolproof way of moving into a state of Deep Calm at the same time as you derive pleasure . . .

I'm referring to massage.

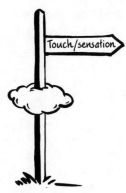

Massage is a powerful way of eliminating many of the harmful effects of stress from the body and, as such, has much to recommend it. More importantly, however, massage is one of those activities that takes almost every person into a state of Deep Calm without requiring any effort whatsoever on their part. Its benefits are cumulative – and someone else expends all the effort.

When you consider that an hour of massage or reflexology costs about the same as a night out on the town, these therapies can be viewed as very accessible calming activities.

I commend massage to you as a highly desirable part of your over-all calming program – a part that can be extraordinarily useful as well as pleasurable. Unfortunately, it will not be something most people can indulge in every day. This is a simple fact of economics or masseur willingness. It is for this reason that I recommend a process of self-massage. It is not for everyone, and it will have no appeal to those who are uncomfortable with their bodies, but it works. And, for those who master the initial stages of the technique, it has significant possibilities.

- Find a warm, quiet, dimly lit place where you will not be disturbed. Remove your clothes and relax on a soft bath towel. Devote a couple of minutes to listening to your breathing and becoming comfortable with your surroundings.

- Tell yourself you have all the time in the world.

- Take a bottle of almond oil. If you like, add a few drops of your favourite relaxing oils (up to 12 drops in 100 ml). Choose no more than three oils from lavender, ylang ylang, rose, orange blossom, sandalwood, geranium, bergamot, neroli, basil and patchouli. If necessary, sit a bottle of this oil blend in tepid water so it warms to body temperature.

- Slowly oil your body, taking care to cover the surface of legs, feet, arms, neck, face, shoulders – in fact, every place you can comfortably reach.

- Now begin to massage each part of your body: slowly, methodically, concentrating your full attention on wherever your hands touch your body. It is important to do this as slowly as possible, since you want to draw out this process for 20–30 minutes. It is not necessary to pummel knotted muscles or work on your aches and pains. This is a process of concentration – where you fill your attention with the sensation of the surface of your hand massaging the surface of other parts of your body.

- Be conscious of what it feels like through the sensation in your hand.

- And be conscious of what it feels like through the sensation of your hand coming into contact with another surface of your body.

- Slowly, methodically, calmly.

The purpose of Strokes of Calm is simply to occupy the senses so completely that your mind is stilled, and your thoughts come to rest. The physical aspect of this exercise should be given no more prominence than listening to your breathing or reciting a meaningless phrase over and over – it has no inherent purpose other than to occupy your attention to the exclusion of all other thought or sensations.

Strokes of Calm is well worth a try. Who knows what you might discover about yourself . . .

A Vision of Calm

At some time you have probably had the experience of sitting in front of an open fire on a cold night, staring into the flames.

And, as you sat there warming yourself, staring into the flickering flames, you suddenly became aware that you'd drifted off into another world . . . a world where there were no time pressures, no responsibilities . . . where you could just be.

At peace.

A Vision of Calm is a reflection of that experience.

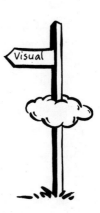

Some people find this technique every bit as easy as it appears. Others struggle with it. It's worth experimenting with it a couple of times to see which category you belong to.

To begin with, choose some sort of restful visual element that you can focus on, uninterrupted, for 20–30 minutes. Consider a burning candle, a tank of tropical fish, a lava lamp, or a fireplace or campfire. (You may find that, in the early stages, a real fire is not suitable if it crackles or demands your attention.)

Alternatively, you could choose a static and less hypnotic image such as a single flower in a vase, a reflection in a polished doorknob, a mandala or any religious icon you feel an affinity with.

The objective is to focus on this object and use all of its visual information to overwhelm your other senses – so that no other thoughts can co-exist. When you do that, your mind will gradually come to rest (that is, open up).

- When you have decided on the focus of this exercise, ease yourself into a comfortable chair before it, or sit on the floor.

- Tell yourself you have all the time in the world.

- Just relax, listening to the sound of your breathing. Listen for 2 minutes.

- Now bring your attention to the object, noting all its visual characteristics, without thinking too much about it. Make no judgements, no assessments, simply observe.

- Without moving your eyes, widen your peripheral vision. (Your vision may go a little blurry, or your eyes watery, but this is nothing to worry about.) Do not stare, and allow your eyes to blink normally.

- Keep observing the object until you feel familiar with it.

- Keep observing until it fills your mind, without your having to think about it.

- When you feel there is nothing else about it to observe, keep observing; you are just reaching the starting point of this exercise.

- When thoughts come, or your attention wanders, pay them no heed. Simply return your attention to the observing as soon as you feel comfortable about doing so.

After a while, you will no longer be aware of the object at all – even though you are focused on it and it is the only thing occupying your attention.

When this happens, you will be experiencing Deep Calm.

Looking Out From the Centre

Instead of searching for your calm centre by looking inwards, you will find so much more can be achieved by looking outwards.

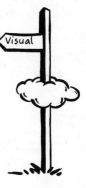

First you assume your calm centre exists. It then becomes the starting point of your experience, rather than the end point.

So, with this in mind, let's explore a technique for viewing the world from your own unique centre. What follows will allow you to do it in a visual way.

The first step is the same as for a Vision of Calm.

- Choose some sort of restful visual element that you can gaze upon, uninterrupted, for 20–30 minutes.

- Tell yourself you have all the time in the world.

- Relax for a couple of minutes, listening to the sound of your breathing.

- Bring your attention to the object, noting its visual elements, without thinking too much about it.

- Without moving your eyes, widen your peripheral vision.

- Now, without moving your eyes or changing your focus, allow your *perspective* to change. Try to imagine seeing what you're see-ing in front of you – not *with* your eyes, but from *behind* your eyes. In other words, try to view the object from inside your head somewhere, so that you're aware of your eyes as well as what they're seeing.

- Next, imagine hearing whatever sounds there are around you, not with your ears, but from *inside* your ears. Be aware of your ears as well as what they're hearing.

- Then, we come to the things you can feel – your back against the chair, your feet on the floor, the breeze on your face. Imagine you're feeling not with the skin of your body, but with the flesh *inside* your body. Be aware of your flesh, as well as what it's feeling.

- Do these three things: seeing, hearing, feeling – from *within* your body rather than *with* your body – and you'll find yourself slipping into a deeper and deeper state of relaxation.

Maintain all of these sensations until you no longer have to think about anything, and are simply centred and aware.

The Calm Journey

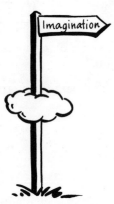

Now we come to the method that I believe is the most powerful of them all. It uses the imagination.

You've heard of guided imagery – when a moderator, either in person or on tape, takes you on a narrated journey into a deeply relaxed, absolutely tranquil place. This all happens inside your head. You go along with the imagery until you stop thinking about what is being described and simply begin to experience it.

Many meditation schools use this same technique.

Before we go any further, I want you to take a deep breath and recall one moment in your past when you felt deeply relaxed, totally at peace.

Or maybe it's a tranquil experience that took place only in your imagination: on an isolated South Pacific island or a mountain in Nepal; diving with whales off Newfoundland or skiing on the snowy slopes of the Swiss Alps; at sunrise in a Zimbabwean game reserve, in the wide open Australian Outback or in a Hindu temple in Bali; or perhaps being cradled in your mother's arms as a baby.

Or maybe it was just a nice warm bath you enjoyed a few nights back. It doesn't matter. All that matters is that you bring to mind a time when you felt, or would have felt, completely calm and relaxed.

If you can't think of one in the next few seconds, close this book for a couple of minutes until one comes to mind. Alternatively, invent your own; there is no necessity for this experience to be one you have savoured before.

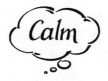

- Find yourself a quiet place where you can sit and reflect on an experience, without interruption, for 20–30 minutes. This is going to be a journey where you can take your time, and enjoy every moment, knowing you can return at any time if you become uncomfortable in any way.

- Remove your wristwatch and place it somewhere out of sight, out of mind. Where you're going, there are no time restrictions, no deadlines, no pressures. Only peace. Pleasure. Fulfilment. And all the time in the world.

- In the back of your mind now is an experience from some relaxed place in your past or your imagination. In this place you felt calm, secure and totally at peace with the world.

- Once you can recall that feeling, you will automatically find yourself beginning to move back into that experience – maybe not in a completely obvious way, but as a subtle relaxed state that you may or may not notice beginning to move through your body. Try not to pay attention to this – it is just a natural part of the process I'm going to tell you about.

- Just think about the experience. Close your eyes and slowly begin to imagine what this place looked like. What hue is the sky? What is the texture of the ground surface? What about the tone of the light? Warm? Cool? Sunrise? Sunset? Don't try to force the image, just let it come if it's going to, and observe it when it does. It is not important that you can see this image, only that you can *imagine* yourself seeing it.

- Soon you will find that it is easy to imagine being at this peaceful, relaxed place. Now that you can do that, imagine you can see yourself in this place. How relaxed do you look? What is the expression on your face? How relaxed is your posture, the way you hold your hands? What are you wearing?

- Now that you can imagine yourself being there, imagine actually *experiencing* being there: looking out at the world through your own eyes; seeing the tranquil, peaceful surroundings with your own eyes.

- And now that you can see this peaceful world around you, pay attention to what you can *hear*. What sound is the breeze making? Is there a running stream or lapping waves nearby? Distant birds, perhaps? What about your own breathing – can you hear how relaxed the sound of your own breath is as it comes and goes? Slowly, deeply, peacefully . . . Your breathing will be slowing down right now, simply because you're imagining this experience. Imagine how relaxed it will be when you can imagine it for real . . .

- And now that you can see the sights, and hear the sounds that surround you, turn your attention to the things you can *feel*. Can you feel the temperature of the sun on your face? The sand or snow beneath your feet? Is there a breeze blowing on your back?

- And, now that you're completely calm and carefree, can you feel how that relaxation affects your facial muscles? How relaxed your hands feel? And your stomach muscles? The complete lack of tension, and the hint of a smile on your face . . .

There's no need for me to continue this any further. You can easily see how 20–30 minutes of this fantasy could take you into another, tranquil world. A world of Deep Calm. Just by using your imagination.

Can it really be as easy as that?

We've been trained to think that nothing great in life comes easily, and that profound states are the hardest to come by. I wish to put that argument to rest. Being calm, enjoying the pleasure of being calm, is quite easy to achieve. All it takes is the right frame of mind, and a few simple techniques.

The Step 3 techniques we have just covered will help you achieve this.

The reason I have given you a choice of techniques is so that you can find the one or ones that best suit your temperament and personality. I have not provided this range so you can flit from one to another, and amuse yourself by trying something different every day. (Although if you choose to do so, that is your choice.)

Repetition and familiarity are the goals.

You should derive pleasure and satisfaction from using these techniques almost from the beginning – as soon as you are familiar with how they're meant to work. If your brain hurts, or you feel uncomfortable performing any of them, this is probably because you're rushing things; or your expectations are too high; or you're using the wrong technique. In most cases, the cause will be one of the first two, although you will probably be inclined to blame the third.

Impatience is an issue we always have to contend with. We live in an overstimulated world of instant solutions. The very notion of sitting around doing virtually nothing is anathema to many of us. Yet, this is the luxury of what I am proposing – that you *can* sit around doing virtually nothing and derive pleasure from it.

Kick off your shoes.
Take off your wristwatch.
Forget about all the pressures and responsibilities
of your everyday life.
You have all the time in the world.
And just relax.
Take it easy, do virtually nothing for 20–30 minutes.
You deserve it.
It is your right.
It will help you become a better human being.
The benefits will multiply over time.

The next cause of discomfort or irritation is expectation.

Many years ago I was asked to write a small meditation book for an Indian teacher. She was in her late sixties, in poor health, and was depending on this book to summarise her meditation teachings for her disciples. It was a priority in her life.

Not long after I started writing it, one of my older books unexpectedly became flavour of the month again and I was lured back onto the speaking circuit. Her book became less of a priority to me.

Later, with her book now months overdue, I went to see her, armed with apologies and excuses. In spite of her need for the book, there was no sign of this in her face. Quite the contrary. She smiled – with neither approval nor disapproval – as if what I had explained was just a pleasantry. I was expecting her to say something like, 'That's okay, I understand business comes first', but she said nothing.

'Were you expecting me to be late?' I asked.

'I expect nothing,' she replied. After she explained that she expected nothing in all facets of her life, I understood the beauty of her philosophy. Not only did it remove all pressure from her relationships and transactions, but it allowed her to live in the moment – something we all recognise as an ideal, but find difficult to achieve.

If you can apply this philosophy to your methods of approaching Deep Calm, every step along the way will bring its own rewards. There are no experiences you must compare yours with. There are no benchmarks. There are no finite outcomes or expectations in using any of the techniques we have covered.

All there is is a process. A state you can enjoy all the way along the path to Deep Calm, whether you believe you have arrived there or not.

Even though I have been describing Deep Calm
as an objective, it is not.
It is a state that can only exist when you are not
conscious of its existence. If you consciously seek it,
you will never find it.
It arrives when you are totally involved in the process of
finding it.
You will know you found it only after you have found it.

The third possibility, that you are using the wrong technique, is one you can only understand through experimentation. In all likelihood, though, you will intuitively make the right choices; if you trust your subconscious or your intuition, you will easily identify the ideal technique or techniques for you.

The pleasure of your company

The Step 3 techniques are designed to be part of your daily routine. If you think of them as a discipline or a chore, you will limit their effectiveness. But when you view them as an escape, a pleasure, an indulgence, their benefits will grow exponentially.

In my earlier books, I advocated a practice that will enrich your life. I call it Self Time. A time to set aside *each day* to do absolutely nothing, for simply being. For escaping the pressures of day-to-day life. For luxuriating in the pleasure of your own company. For discovering what good company you can be!

It is a fact that most people today allow themselves very little quality 'alone time', where they sit by themselves and do nothing – no reading, thinking about work, listening to the radio or trying to catch up on sleep. Generally, they would consider Self Time a waste of time. They believe that if they have a free hour, that time should be spent 'productively' – watching the news, catching up with correspondence. This is not only misdirected thinking, it is 100 percent wrong.

Self Time is not a squandering of time, it is a time enhancer. It makes the rest of your day more fulfilling. It allows you to do more in your life, to be able to approach the other activities of your day with increased focus, application and enjoyment. And all it takes is 20–30 minutes each day. Or twice a day if you want to enrich your life even further.

You *can* fit it in! You *do* have the time. Your work, your partner, or your children *will* allow you this space – even if you have to rise earlier to achieve it. Don't worry; the techniques I have given you will more than compensate for half an hour of sleep, as far as feeling rested is concerned.

After you adjust your perspective – just a little – so that you see Self Time as a time-enhancer rather than a time-waster, everything begins to change. You will suddenly see this as *your* time. A pleasurable time. A time of supreme indulgence, when you can shrug off all your responsibilities and pressures, and just relax. You will feel positive about using this time in such a way because you know it is doing good for you. And you will feel no guilt at taking this time for yourself because you know that the effort will repay itself, over and over again, in other areas of your life.

The above techniques are designed to occupy your Self Time. Make the decision to create this time for yourself, and the practice of Step 3 techniques will never seem like a chore. They will seem like the most indulgent, pleasurable moments of your day. And the more you practise them, the more effective they become.

The making of habit

Earlier in this book we covered how habits are formed: how, by following the same thought processes, you create well-worn 'thought paths' (neural pathways) in your brain. All the learning processes in your life – simple sums, spelling, riding a bicycle – are created by establishing these thought paths. These can assume either the elegance of learning, or the compulsion of habit. Either way, you can make this phenomenon work in your favour.

If you make a habit of going to your calm centre, and practising Deep Calm, you will establish a powerful, calm thought path. The more you use it, the better established that path becomes. And the faster you can move to this wonderful, peaceful state known as Deep Calm.

There is another benefit in this process. The more you practise – easing into a tranquil, carefree state by following this thought path – the more you begin to associate that beautiful relaxed feeling with just *starting* down the path.

This is known as a Programmed Conditioned Response (PCR), and was first identified in Pavlov's dog experiments. A specific response (in our case, feeling calm, happy and tranquil) is associated with an apparently unrelated stimulus (listening to the sound of your breathing). PCRs work so powerfully that they are at the root of most phobias, fetishes, irrational fears, and inexplicable likes and dislikes. It is a PCR that makes some people squirm at the sound of a dentist's drill, become sexually aroused at the sight of red patent leather shoes, or get embarrassed when asked a question in front of an audience.

But you can also use PCRs to positive effect. For example, if you've been using the Breath of Calm on a regular basis, you'll soon begin to associate the sensation of peace and deep relaxation (a PCR) with the sound of your breathing.

I have been doing this so long myself that, simply by concentrating on the sound of *one* deep breath, I am well down the path to feeling very calm and peaceful. That's all it takes. Just listen to one deep intake of breath and a sense of calm follows.

This is more than just a feeling. Accompanying that sense of calm is a change in physiology – where one can move from being physically tense to physically relaxed in a few short moments. In other words, instant calm.

You might be able to imagine how powerful such an ability could be in your life.

Step 3 and beyond

The Step 3 techniques we've just explored have immeasurably more potential than they might at first seem to have. I have formulated them as simple exercises that will fit into your everyday life. And while I have deliberately underplayed their scope, what you have in those few techniques is the basis of *all* meditation practice.

If you've spent years studying a particular method of meditation, you may baulk at that assertion. Some meditation teachers would say these are merely the *techniques* of classic meditation, not the content or even the intention. Even if this is true, it does not lessen their potential.

Indeed, I would go so far as to make you this guarantee: if you devote as much dedication and practice to my techniques as any traditional meditation school would ask you to devote to theirs, the psychological and physiological results will be very similar. Very similar.

This is not to suggest that years of training in yoga or Chi Kung would not teach you much more. Of course they would. Similarly, I make no spiritual claims in respect of the above methods – this is the province of the traditional schools. But I can assure you that, with dedication and practice, the techniques of Deep Calm will be just as effective from a temporal point of view as any classic meditation method.

Later in this book, you will discover how to use these Step 3 techniques as a springboard to further development if your interest turns from the temporal to the spiritual. Because now that you know the path to Deep Calm, and how to access your calm centre at will, all things suddenly become possible. In spirituality, healing, prosperity, happiness, relationships . . . indeed, in almost any area you can think of.

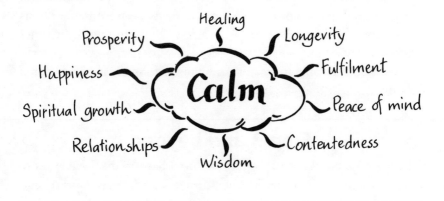

Step 4

Have you ever been on an extended vacation – say 6 or 7 weeks?

Before you embark on it, you spend several weeks in anticipation: planning, preparing, daydreaming. From time to time, you find yourself slipping into 'vacation mode' before your duties, or another person, bring you back to the here and now.

This equates with Step 1.

Then you go on vacation. For the first week, you think: 'This is fantastic. So relaxing. Such a contrast to normal working life.' You think you are relaxed, that your everyday life is a million miles away, and that this is as good as it gets.

This equates with Step 2.

In the second week you start to get twitchy. You feel you should be doing something more. Some people describe this as working the stress out of your system. More accurately, I suspect, it is a necessary act of preparation for the weeks ahead. Because in the third week you suddenly start to unwind. You feel comfortable sitting around doing nothing. It doesn't bother you if nothing interesting happens each day. Time no longer seems important. You are relaxed. Moreover, you are not conscious of being relaxed – you simply are.

This equates with Step 3.

The next step arrives without fanfare. You are simply not aware of it. Time is forgotten. You may find yourself having moments of inspiration, remembering things you thought you'd long since forgotten, being more intuitive with others and more open in new situations – or you may not notice anything much different. If you do not notice, it is because you don't think to notice; you simply take those things for granted.

When you are most aware of these restful and intuitive qualities within yourself is when the vacation is over and you return to your everyday life.

On your first day back at work, you notice everyone is speaking much faster than sounds normal to you. The motives of the office politicians are more transparent to you. Aspects of your job seem trivial and unnecessarily complex. When your workmates hurriedly describe things to you, you become conscious of the shorthand of their language. You seek elaboration of points they expect you to grasp immediately – you do this, not because you fail to understand, but because you're endeavouring to slow down the pace of communication.

You do other things as well. You blank out the negatives, the criticisms, the sarcasm. You purposely speak more slowly, move more slowly. You cling to the restful state you have been enjoying, that you thought you'd brought back with you, in the naïve hope that you can extend it, that you can prevent it from ebbing away. But by the end of the day, you are back to 'normal' and all of those feelings are little more than a memory.

In the days before you returned to work, you were enjoying a state that equates with Step 4. You were not conscious of it, you just accepted it as natural. In this state, your thinking abilities were significantly sharper, more refined and more creative than in your normal work-intensive mode. But you did not notice. Nor did you notice that you could access these abilities without conscious effort, and without interruption to your state of inner calm.

Whereas in Steps 2 and 3 you were conscious of becoming more relaxed (and probably conscious of your moments of inspiration or intuition), in Step 4 these things became integral, or holistic. They were simply part of you; they just happened.

Step 4 is not normally something you can effect of your own accord. It is the product of time and practice. In this state, you no longer have to suppress conscious thoughts to enjoy Deep Calm. You can enjoy direct access to your subconscious and unconscious, become more intuitive and wise, direct your health, enhance all of your natural abilities, and be able to realise your fullest potential.

This is an ongoing state of enhanced awareness. It is the result of many years' experience of Deep Calm. It is *not* a mystical state. It is real and measurable. I have seen it many times in EEGs of the brain-wave patterns of yogis and martial arts masters. I have experienced it myself (on a temporary basis).

Step 4 is a unique mental state where beta-intense frequencies can co-exist with the other frequencies that are normally present only in the meditative state. In this instance, the beta-intense frequencies are not representative of a tense state of mind, but simply of mental alertness and an active conscious mind . . . *at the same time as you are deeply relaxed and in touch with your unconscious!*

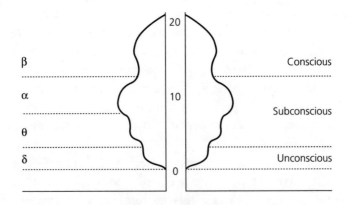

The Step 4 brainwave state

On the surface, this may seem impossible. You may think there could not be many people in this world capable of existing in such a state. But such people do exist. It is possible for most of us to exist in this state for long periods of time, if not on a permanent basis. And it all stems from regular use of Deep Calm and visits to your calm centre. Twice a day.

Twice a day? You don't think you can manage that? Yes you can! Remember, you have all the time in the world.

So far, you've discovered that:

- **Being calm is a choice.**

- **It is easy to become calm – at will.**

- **Your greatest power and your maximum potential come from your calm centre.**

- **There are many paths to your calm centre and the experience of Deep Calm.**

- **You can choose from several Step 2 exercises that can help you to relax.**

- **You can then choose from several Step 3 exercises that can take you to your calm centre and the experience of Deep Calm.**

- **From this Deep Calm state, you can achieve extraordinary things.**

7

FROM CALM
COMES POWER

*Once you know how to attain the
state of Deep Calm, you can
achieve anything you set your mind
to – just by applying a couple of
simple formulae . . .*

Everything you have read so far is designed to illustrate two things:

(i)   that it is easy to access a profoundly calm state (Deep Calm) that can enhance your health and attitude as much as your peace of mind;

(ii) that in spite of how you've been conditioned and educated, in spite of what you've been taught was possible or impossible, there *is* a way you can seize control of your life and fortunes, and dictate their course.

The first part is easy. If you've been experimenting with the techniques we've covered so far, you will understand just how easy these are.

The second part may require a little faith. However, like all opportunities in life, there are those who will grasp it by the scruff of the neck and use it to enrich their lives; and there are those who will stand back, wondering, 'Why not me?'. . . until the moment passes.

Now we're going to explore how to use the deeper levels of relaxation that you find at your calm centre – Deep Calm – so you will intuitively know the most beneficial directions, decisions and actions to take in life. Whether we're referring to health, spirituality, career planning, relationships or just peace of mind, no other person will ever be in a position to know your ideal path as well as you do. Experts can make suggestions, teachers and learned people can guide you, but only you will know what the right answers are for you.

At this moment, you have no way of knowing that this can be so. Or, worse still, you may consciously think it *cannot* be so – in your case. That's okay. That's how most people initially view these skills. As long as you are prepared to approach the second half of this book with an open mind, your own experience will provide all the proof you require.

Even though you may not yet know this on a conscious level, subconsciously you are well down the path to using these skills for your own enrichment.

Success beyond calm

Success means different things to different people.

If you currently manage a large corporation, your idea of success might be global expansion and 10 million stock options each year; but if you haven't worked for 2 years, your idea of success could be finding a satisfying job of any type.

If you're a happy, relaxed person with plenty of spare time on your hands, your idea of success could be spiritual enlightenment through meditation; but if you're in a poor relationship, a nervous wreck at the end of your tether, your idea of success may be just finding a little peace of mind.

Every time you achieve something significant in life – anything that is out of the ordinary when compared with *your* normal, every-day standards – you tend to adopt a certain procedure. Most people would describe this as 'working harder' or 'being more focused', but usually it will be a little more complicated than this.

The Success Formula

If A equals success, then the formula is: A = X + Y + Z; where X is work, Y is play, Z is keep your mouth shut.

Albert Einstein

For 11 years now I have been studying people you would normally describe as successful. These are people who, by most conventional standards, have produced extraordinary levels of beneficial change in their lives.

The questions on my mind were: Did they share any particular attributes? If they did, could this be formularised in any meaningful way? I was intrigued by the possibility that there could be such a thing as a 'success formula'.

I now know that such a formula exists. Moreover, it is exactly the same formula that you apply – albeit unconsciously – when you achieve things in your everyday life.

Almost everyone I could classify as a self-made success intuitively employed this formula. It applied equally to healers and househusbands as it did to world-champion athletes, businesspeople, therapists, academics, potters, scientists, writers, artists and one-man surfboard manufacturers. (I have excluded those who attributed their success to luck, inheritance, privilege or divine intervention.) Also included in this group were people who survived 'incurable' illnesses, or overcame great physical adversity. They, too, intuitively used a formula such as this.

I want to share it with you now. It is presented as an equation for no other reason than that I've been using it this way for years in my lectures. It requires no understanding of maths, so if you were starting to feel mathematically intimidated, just relax.

Relax.

$$(M+B+F)^i = C$$

This simple formula places success – of any type – within your reach. So, whether your objective is to cure yourself of an illness, win a new job, make your partner happy, set up an eye hospital in Angola, make a million, or just be a happy person with all the time in the world, this formula will help you to achieve it.

What does it take?

The C in this formula is for Consequence: the outcome or end result. I like to think of the word 'consequence' as having much more power than 'outcome'. To me, an outcome sounds like an eventuality that you may, or may not, have played a role in; a consequence, on the other hand, is the product of effort and implies a responsibility. Even if what you are seeking is a process (such as becoming happy) rather than a finite result, as far as this formula is concerned it can be defined as a Consequence.

M is for Motivation. Why, and how badly, do you want to achieve the Consequence you nominate for yourself? Why is it important to you? How much are you prepared to invest in order to attain it?

It is next to impossible to achieve anything of note without Belief, the B of this formula. How often have you observed people with all the right qualifications and resources who, through lack of belief in themselves or the possibility of success, never achieve anything they set out to achieve?

Most of the motivational experts would have taken your money and sent you home by now. If you have the motivation and the belief, or conviction, they say, you have everything you need.

They are incorrect.

You have everything you need to be a second-rate salesperson. But to transform this motivation into something that will enrich your life and overcome adversity, you need something more: Focus, F.

Effort vs Consequence

If I asked you right now what it takes to do well in any particular area, you would probably say effort. A great amount of effort. So on one side of our formula is the 'effort'.

The other side represents the Consequence or goal. The effort always has to balance the Consequence.

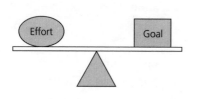

To achieve anything worthwhile in life, your effort usually has to be equal to the goal or the consequence you seek. Small goals require small effort, while extreme goals require extreme effort. No surprises here.

The 'effort' parts of our equation are Motivation, Belief and Focus. For any given Consequence, you need a combination of these elements. For a Consequence that is beyond the norm (meaning what you believe is the norm), you will need even more Motivation, Belief and Focus. A greater effort.

This is not radical thinking; it is a fundamental of life. The bigger the goal, the harder you have to work towards attaining it.

We could have left the formula there: $M + B + F = C$.

Applying the formula

According to this formula, you do not have to have equal amounts of Motivation, Belief and Focus. You could, for example, achieve your Consequence by applying an additional measure of Motivation – thus requiring less Belief and reduced Focus. Or, you could achieve the same result by having an unshakeable Belief – so that less

Motivation and Focus are required. As long as the effort side is equal to the goal side.

Effort	Goal
M = Motivation **B** = Belief **F** = Focus	**C** = Consequence

All things being equal.

Aha, you see the flaw. All things in life are not equal. Sometimes the odds are stacked against you. Sometimes you want things that are considered beyond the reach of people like yourself. Sometimes your ambition far outweighs your known capabilities or opportunities. Sometimes the issue is so big, so important, that all commonsense and proportion flies out the window.

For issues such as these it may simply not be possible to achieve what you want to achieve by applying the necessary levels of Motivation, Belief or Focus – no matter how much of these you can muster.

So this brings us to the fifth element of our equation, **i**.

i is for a range of calm intangibles that include I (you), imagination, intuition. More precisely, it is the Inspiration part of our formula, the 'How?'.

i is the magic ingredient; it creates a multiplier effect. You take all of the 'effort' elements – Motivation, Belief and Focus – and amplify them to the power of **i**. This transforms a fairly straightforward formula into something with virtually unlimited potential.

$$(M+B+F)^i = C$$

The beauty of this formula is that it allows you to choose any Consequence you desire. This can be as big, as hopeful, and as extravagant as you dare to dream of. There is no limit as to how bold you can be in this decision. Indeed, if ever there was a time when you had no excuse for not dreaming the big dreams, it is now.

Choose any Consequence or goal your imagination can handle. The only thing to bear in mind is that the more ambitious the Consequence (C), the more you must compensate with your Motivation (M), Belief (B) and Focus (F). The bigger the goal, the more of these 'effort' elements you will require.

For example, 'I want to be Managing Director by Friday' would be a huge goal for most people. It is possible. But for you to achieve it in that time frame would usually require an immense amount of motivation, belief and focus. Providing you can furnish these in sufficient quantity, you should theoretically be able to achieve the goal. (Life is never as simple as that, of course. This is why i assumes such importance in this equation.)

Here's how it works . . .

M

Motivation is the area of personal development that has received more than its deserved share of prominence in recent years. This has largely been due to the proliferation of high-profile motivational speakers, and the desire of corporate heads to motivate the troops.

The reason there are so many of these speakers is a combination of show business and career paths. How else can a footballer get an adrenalin boost once he's past 35? How else can prominent military or corporate generals get their leadership juices flowing when they're no longer required by the organisations they once led? How else are adventurers meant to occupy their time while raising funds for their next expedition?

And the reason these people are in demand is simply that today's corporate leaders often fail in their most basic of duties: to inspire and motivate. So when these highly paid speakers appear at seminars, salespeople and business executives queue by the thousands to be fired up by carefully crafted sporting or adventure stories, which serve as metaphors for a range of corporate virtues such as determination and team spirit.

You know the drill: a dramatic story of human endeavour, a fervent message, then everyone leaves the room motivated. For about 90 minutes. After that, most of the audience will remember the anecdote, but will have forgotten the relevance. A couple of days later, and even the anecdote will have been forgotten.

Motivational courses do not fare much better. According to one survey, attendees of these courses demonstrated an average 'decay factor', characterised by declining interest or memory of the event, of between 1 and 4 days after returning to work.

There is only one person in the world who can really motivate you. That's you.

So what is motivation?

Motivation is the 'Why?' in life. When you decide there is something you really want, motivation is what provides the direction and energy to achieve it. Motivation is what encourages some people to go that little extra distance while others are happy to potter along in their slipstream. Motivation is what allows some people to overcome adversity while others succumb to it. Motivation is what makes and maintains success. And, most attractive of all, motivation is a skill you can learn.

The starting point is recognising the drives that reside within you now, simply because you're a human being. These aim to satisfy your 'survival needs' (hunger, thirst), 'social needs' (sex, maternal instinct) and 'curiosity'.

But wiser people than I have said that all motivations can be narrowed down to two primary drives: obtaining pleasure and avoiding pain. This has been proposed, then elaborated on, for centuries. It appears in early Buddhist teachings, in the writings of Sigmund Freud and even in the Nobel Peace Prize acceptance speech of the Dalai Lama, Tenzin Gyatso: 'No matter what part of the world we come from, we are all basically the same human beings. We all seek happiness and try to avoid suffering.'

Knowing this is one of the keys to your motivation. Obtaining pleasure, avoiding pain. One of these forces is more powerful than the other. Can you guess which?

Here's a test. Answer the following questions truthfully:

(i)   Can you run 100 metres in 11 seconds?

(ii) If I offered you $100,000 to run 100 metres in 11 seconds, do you think you could come close to it?

If you answered 'no' to the first question, chances are you'd have to answer 'no' to the second. The offer of a prize (that is, pleasure) is usually insufficient motivation to succeed.

But think about this scenario:

You're walking through a nice, quiet field. There's a noise. You turn, and see a massive, snorting, longhorn steer charging out of the trees towards you. Now would you come close to running 100 metres in 11 seconds?

Of course you would. Because, masochism aside, avoiding pain is a much stronger motivation than obtaining pleasure. The reason I'm pointing this out is that negative motivation (avoidance of pain) can be a great limiter in life. You want to avoid the pain of failure more than you want the pleasure of success; you want to avoid the pain of making the wrong decision by making no decision at all; you want to avoid the pain of missing out on a party rather than enjoy the pleasure of having an hour to meditate and be by yourself.

Making motivations positive

This is not difficult. It can be achieved by making a game of the process – the process of positive substitution. Be on the lookout for negative sentiments and perspectives; when they arise, immediately substitute a positive that achieves the same end.

To enhance this game, invest in a hard-covered notebook (the hard cover will make it seem more important). On each spread, write '–' on the left, and '+' on the right. Each time a negative arises, see how creative you can be in composing a more compelling positive to replace it with. Although this will sometimes seem difficult, it's worth persevering because out of this process there comes a transforming view of what's going on in your life and what can be made of it.

After some time of this, positive substitutions can become a lifetime habit – not just in how you motivate yourself but in all of life's activities.

It is not easy to remove negative motivations. As you know from the third of the Calm Centre's Nine Mental Powers, the Power of Substitution, the only way of consciously changing a thought, habit or behaviour is to substitute another. This is why you need to fill your mind with positive motivations. You must be *overwhelmingly* positive in the thoughts, words, attitudes and actions that relate to what you aspire to.

The process of building positive motivation can be enjoyable in its own right. It's a simple, self-indulgent fantasy. In reality, it is more than this, but let's treat it as something light and pleasurable.

Take a notebook and pencil to a quiet place where you will not be disturbed. Sit quietly for a few minutes, close your eyes and listen to the sound of your breathing. Tell yourself you have all the time in the world.

When you feel deeply relaxed, think about the Consequence you have chosen for yourself.

Imagine yourself having attained this goal. Loved, cured, rich, happy, well, slim, making a difference – whatever it is you have chosen. Try to imagine every last detail of your life once you have attained this: what you are wearing; what people are saying to you, or about you; what you are seeing when you're in that position; what you are hearing; what you *feel* about it all.

Now, open your eyes and write down the very first thing that comes to mind about *why* you need to achieve this goal.

Sit quietly for a few minutes thinking about this 'need'. That is your first motivation.

You can repeat this exercise many times (preferably on different days), each time writing down why you need to achieve this goal. After a few days of this, recording and thinking about all these reasons, your positive motivations should far outweigh the negative.

They can because they think they can.
Virgil

In studying the people I considered to have produced extraordinary levels of beneficial change in their lives, the first question to resolve was: were these extraordinary people? Did they have special skills, or education, or natural abilities that set them apart from ordinary folk like you and me?

The answer was a resounding no. In fact, if there is one comfort you can immediately take from this it's that talent counts for very little in life. Those who win are seldom the strongest, the best educated or the most intelligent, they're the people who think they can win. It's all in the state of mind.

Whether based on fact or fallacy, belief is remarkably empowering. Indeed, in almost all aspects of your life, what you believe is more meaningful than what can be proved to be true. An assessment or opinion may be completely incorrect, yet if you believe it to be correct it has exactly the same effect as if it were. Conversely, if you believe something to be incorrect, it might as well be incorrect.

Your version of reality is created by what you believe. Regardless of what our scientists, politicians and educators contend, belief is more powerful than fact. And when it comes to succeeding in any area: belief outperforms fact every time; and conviction outperforms talent most of the time.

If you've ever done martial arts and progressed to the showy stage of smashing bricks and blocks of timber with your bare hands, you will have discovered something remarkable about the nature of belief. When you believe in your capabilities, when you have absolute faith in your power, when you commit your fist to being just a small distance on the *other* side of the brick, the 'impossible' is quite easily achieved. But, if just a glimmer of doubt intrudes, you end up with a fractured hand.

One interesting study compared confidence and raw talent in children, to see which attribute produced the better result over the long term. In almost all cases, the confident children (those who were identified by their strong faith in their own ability) outperformed the talented ones (those who were identified by talent alone) in the longer term. The confident children were more curious, more willing to participate, and more persistent – and as the years passed, they excelled. The talented, but less confident ones, performed nowhere near as well.

You've probably seen examples of this yourself. How often do executives who believe they are in control end up in control? How often do tennis players who believe they can win end up winning? The fact that you believe you are capable of a certain performance is usually all it takes to ensure you attain it. Fact and reality have little to do with it. *Feelings* have everything to do with it.

If you *feel* you are capable, you are capable. If you *feel* you are succeeding, you almost certainly are succeeding. Because as we know from the Nine Mental Powers, if you feel a certain way about something, your subconscious accepts it as reality, and immediately sets about making it real. So to enhance your belief about achieving any Consequence you define, you have to *feel* that you are capable and that it is possible.

I admit that my scientist friends shudder when I speak about 'feeling'. The concept of being guided by feeling as opposed to knowing is anathema to them. But I am not advocating you abandon knowledge; I am advocating that you allow your intuition – which is really only a manifestation of your subconscious knowledge – to guide you as well.

Information plus intuition is a powerful combination.

What you think becomes   Thoughts create beliefs in the same way that feelings do. What you think about, becomes. If you think about how hopeless life is, life will be hopeless. If you think about how good life is, life will be good. If you think loving thoughts, you will feel and will attract love. If you think about good health and prosperity, you will attract good health and prosperity. Whatever you dwell on becomes self-fulfilling.

There may be the temptation to dismiss this concept as self-help fancy, but there are sound psychological reasons for its effectiveness. The bottom line is this: each person is nothing more than the product of his or her thoughts. At the very earliest age we are taught the thoughts that will limit us, or empower us, for the rest of our lives. These thoughts, or thought patterns, then become our reality.

If person A is taught it's a cold, unfriendly, lonely world out there, they will discover just how cold, unfriendly and lonely the world can be.

If person B is taught that it's a wondrous, love-filled, opportunity-rich world we live in, then they will discover just how wondrous, love-filled and opportunity-rich the world really is.

If both person A and person B walk through identical doors, at the same time, and look out on identical cityscapes, they will see two totally different worlds: person A's will be cold, unfriendly and lonely; person B's will be wondrous, love-filled and opportunity-rich. The same physical world in both cases, but two totally different perceptions of it. And, from the moment they walk out of those doors, their perceptions begin to be transformed into experiences.

A car drives past with its powerful amplifier blasting out an Oasis song, and person A is affronted by the inconsiderate behaviour of playing loud music in public; person B hears only the beautiful music (and the lyric referring to Paul Wilson's *Little Book of Calm*).

They turn the corner and are approached by a paint-splattered, bare-footed young woman. Person A turns away to avoid an unsavoury character; person B listens and makes friends with a prominent young artist.

It has nothing to do with what is real or what logic says *should* be real. Your attitudes and thoughts create your version of reality. And if you want to alter this version of reality in any way – to make it healthier, happier, calmer or more successful – all you have to do is adjust your thoughts or ways of thinking. At first, this might appear to be a daunting task. And all the more so if you've spent the last few years in analysis, talking around deep-seated ways of thinking that were not serving you well. But, in the main, it is quite easy to change thought processes – even those that have been with you since childhood.

The first step is making the decision to change. Make that decision – with conviction – and you're on the way.

The next step could involve any one of several mental techniques described in this book. However, the easiest way to create new beliefs for yourself is by performing one simple ritual: pretence.

For example, if you want to change yourself from a tense, anxious person into one who is calm and relaxed, follow these four steps:

(i) **Analyse.** Note the characteristics of a person who is calm, relaxed and at peace with the world.

(ii) **Imagine.** Imagine yourself as such a person. Note your slow breathing, unhurried speech, relaxed gestures, the hint of a smile.

(iii) **Pretend.** Start pretending you are exactly like the person you are imagining. Be as lavish as you like in your pretence – no-one will notice, only your subconscious.

(iv) **Compound the pretence.** Finally, pretend that others see you as the calm, relaxed person you're pretending to be.

You can believe whatever you'd like to believe about yourself, and achieve whatever you believe you're capable of achieving – it's all a matter of choice and technique.

F

Happiness is nothing more than good health and a bad memory.
Albert Schweitzer

I want to share an exciting, mind-stretching concept with you.

What you see with your very own eyes is not always what is there. Indeed, what you see is usually distorted in some way. Distorted by where you're looking; distorted by your way of looking; possibly even distorted by what you want to see. So, too, with what you hear.

Have you ever noticed how easy it is to misread the mood of a large-scale event that's taking place?

Imagine walking into a large crowd and the first thing you see is five people arguing loudly, a young woman standing off to the side sobbing, and a dozen or so others crowded around looking variously concerned or enjoying the spectacle. How would you be feeling?

Chances are you'd be a little distressed, and your opinion of that event would not be terribly high.

Now let's approach from another angle.

Imagine walking into the same large crowd and the first thing you see is a middle-aged couple, the man tenderly adjusting the collar on the woman's shirt; behind them three people are smiling at a fourth's story; a woman beside you casually comments on the beautiful weather . . . how would you be feeling?

Chances are you'd describe it as nice, or something to that effect.

And, if you were to walk into the same crowd and see three people – one after the other – each of whom gave you the eye and gave your pulse a jolt; then you looked over to the side and a couple were locked in a passionate embrace . . . you'd have a totally different feeling, and a totally different opinion of that crowd.

On each of those three occasions, you walked into the same large crowd of people. Yet the way you felt, and the opinions you formed, were completely different depending on what you focused on. You will be familiar with this experience, because it will have happened to you many times before.

This is the nature of life. How you feel and how you perceive 'reality' depend entirely on where you are looking.

And when someone pronounces that their view of reality is more real than yours – because their perspective is different from yours – they are talking through their hat. Arrogant nonsense. Because 'reality' is endlessly flexible. And reality depends entirely on the perspective and the various biases of the viewer. Or, at least, that is my perspective on reality.

At any given instant, there are billions of linked or independent (depending on your perspective) events taking place around you. Take the room you're sitting in now. There are billions of different elements and forces at play in that very room. How you feel about these things, how they affect your mood, your attitude towards life, and your very life itself, depend entirely on your focus.

If you're at home and your focus is on your present standard of living, you may feel a bit depressed about the peeling paint, the fraying carpet, and the fact that someone as worthy as you has been forced to live in such drab surroundings.

If your focus is on microbiology, you might be alarmed at the deadly cocktail of airborne moulds and viruses swirling about you.

If your focus is on your waistline, you might not notice a single thing outside yourself.

And if your focus is on the wonder and beauty of life – because you met this beautiful man at a party last night – you might marvel at the artistic sensitivity and delicacy that went into a tiny water-colour on the wall.

In each instance, the same person in the same surroundings. The only difference is a matter of perspective. Of focus.

This is as good a time as any for a science joke. Three academics – an astrophysicist, a cosmologist and an archeologist – are on an archeological dig at the base of the Sphinx. Their Egyptian guide points to a magnificent canopy of stars.

'All those stars,' he says, 'you know what that means?'

'It means there are billions of stars in our galaxy,' insists the astrophysicist, 'and potentially billions of galaxies. It means we are insignificant in the grand scheme of things.'

The cosmologist continues: 'We are witnessing events that took place millions of light years ago, and we are just seeing evidence of it now. It means we are physically connected to the past.'

They turn to the archeologist. She takes note of the haze around the moon and says, 'It means we're in for a windy day of digging tomorrow.'

Then all three academics turn to their Egyptian guide: 'And tell us, my good fellow,' sniffs the cosmologist, 'all those pretty stars in the sky. What does it mean to someone like you?'

'It means somebody stole our tent.'

In each instance, the same event: a brilliant night sky. The only difference is a matter of perspective. Of focus. Moreover, it is a focus that we have some control over!

Here we come to one of the big guiding principles of life. For want of a more modest title, let's call it Wilson's Prescription for Focus Choice. It states:

> *As reality is endlessly flexible and variable,*
> *we might as well vary it to suit the ends*
> *we'd like to see.*

All it means is that you adjust your focus on life so that *your* reality is garnished with whatever pleasure, satisfaction and results you desire. Naturally, there are going to be critics of this recommendation. I can almost hear them now.

'That is a prescription for blatant escapism.'

'Life is not meant to be that easy.'

'That's not facing up to reality.'

I suggest you leave it to your critics to face up to their 'reality' if they wish. Let them choose to be unhappy, depressed, tense, or whatever their reality entails, while you 'blindly' get whatever you want out of life . . . being calm, happy, overcoming illness, making a difference in the world around you, even attracting worldly gain, if that is what you want.

I heard an academic recently railing against Walt Disney's manufactured optimism because he presented a world to children that just wasn't real. She went on to describe the 'real' world that children should know about. I, for one, don't want to have any part of the world she described.

Make the choice to focus on the things that will make you feel good and will do you good, and you'll be surprised how quickly the benefits follow.

Broadening the focus

In pre-scientific times, life was easy to understand: Greek philosophers notwithstanding, what could not be explained by direct experience was explained by one of many magical or mystical formulae – often involving the planets, spirits or gods.

The good old Newtonian world of science changed all that: in this world, there was a physical reason for everything, and everything slotted neatly into its place. As a result, life became easier to understand. But the moment we started fooling around with sub-atomic particles (through quantum mechanics), confusion, contradiction and paradox became the order of the day.

What this suggests to me is that the closer we look at any given area, the more restlessness is exposed. And the broader our perspective, the more order and harmony exists.

Not very scientific, I admit – but, hey, it feels good!

How focus helps   The most important consideration in relation to focus is purely a matter of energy efficiency. You only have a certain amount of psychic energy (the total of your mental, physical and spiritual energy) at your disposal at any particular time. You can choose to scatter this energy – by trying to cover several areas at once – or you can concentrate it on one particular area.

It takes no great mental leap to appreciate that concentrating your energy on one particular area improves the result, while scattering your energies across many produces scattered results. You see examples of this time and time again.

If someone thought and spoke from a young age about little else but making a million out of real estate, you just know they're going to make a million out of real estate. Whereas someone who starts out wanting to make a million out of real estate, find a cure for AIDS, write a movie script, climb K2 and become an internationally recognised jazz pianist, stands very little chance of achieving any of them.

The biggest achievements in life require singular focus, at least for part of the time.

If, for example, you are faced with a major health problem that resists conventional treatment, and the Consequence you decide on is a complete recovery, you have a clear-cut choice. You can concentrate on overcoming the problem, applying all your thoughts and energy to this task; or you can carry on as usual, going to work each day, struggling to appear cheery and in control, worrying about your mortgage, trying to reassure your children that you're not depressed or despondent, and hoping that someone or something will intercede and cure you.

What do you think your chances of recovery are?

I'll tell you. They are dramatically improved when you concentrate wholly on the solution.

Dramatically.

C

This brings us, once again, to the Consequence – the end result or outcome of all your efforts. (Please note that the following has been designed with everyday plans, ambitions and decisions in mind. For the major issues in life – those that have long-lasting consequences – you need to go one step further. This is covered in 'Life design' on page 236.)

On being introduced to the Success Formula, many people think that the levels of motivation, belief and focus required are beyond their capabilities. To ensure that you do not entertain such insecurities, I will show you a way of structuring a Consequence so that it stimulates the required levels of the other elements. The way of doing this is to present the Consequence in its most compelling and powerful form – so that it will seem real right from the beginning.

> *Essentially, the more real you can make your*
> *Consequence seem, the easier it is to realise it.*

You know that reality (or at least the reality that relates to you) is endlessly flexible, so the challenge is to design it exactly the way you intend to have it in your Consequence. You'll be pleased to know that this also can be formularised.

To make your Consequence seem real, it must satisfy four requirements – it must be specific, holistic, positive, and based in the present.

Specific There are real things in life and there are abstract concepts. Real things consist of matter and benchmarks; they have dimensions, physical and emotional attributes; sometimes they can be quantified. Abstract concepts, on the other hand, are impossible to quantify and sometimes even difficult to define with any precision.

Real things are infinitely easier to attain.

For this reason, it is much easier to earn a million than it is to be rich. ('A million' is specific – you can imagine what it looks and feels like – whereas 'rich' is non-specific and blurred.) For the same reason, it is much easier to become 'managing director' than it is to become 'successful'. (Managing director is specific, whereas successful can mean any number of things.) And it is easier to find 'calm' than it is to find 'contentment'; easier to 'paint a picture by Friday' than it is 'to be an artist'; easier to get a date with that woman you met in a restaurant than it is to be in a long-lasting relationship.

The more specific something is, the easier it is to achieve.

Get the picture? Keep that thought in mind; we'll come back to it later.

Holistic The second attribute of your Consequence is that it should be holistic. It should be harmonious, not only with your external thoughts and values, but with your secret and not-so-secret needs and values as well.

For example, there's no point in nominating a brilliant career in medicine as your Consequence if all your instincts tell you to manufacture surfboards. Similarly, there's no point in planning a miracle cure with herbal remedies if you secretly believe that only orthodox medicine can work. Any politician will tell you it is much easier to succeed when you work with people's existing belief systems than when you try to create new ones for them.

But what if your belief systems say your objective is impossible?

Fortunately the sections ahead will show you how to *modify* your belief systems in a subtle, non-confronting way.

If, after doing that, your Consequence still does not harmonise with your existing values and belief systems – but is still important to you – there are other options.

Whatever, if you make your Consequence specific and holistic, you are half way to achieving it.

Positive If there's one thing in life you can be sure of, it's that most optimists succeed, whereas *all* pessimists fail.

There have been many clinical studies conducted into how optimism and positive attitudes can affect the prognosis of illnesses. Although few researchers will state for certain that optimism does prolong life for, say, cancer sufferers, they *will* agree that pessimism shortens it.

Even if there was no overwhelming clinical proof that a positive attitude has a positive effect on healing, you should find it easy to accept. Haven't you seen with your own eyes that the healthy people, the successful people, the people with good relationships are invariably positive in their attitude?

Whether you fully accept the power of positive thinking or not, there are many areas where the positive demonstrably outperforms the negative. Positive language is more persuasive, and communicates more effectively than negative language. Positive instructions work more emphatically on the subconscious than negative, which is why hypnotists always couch their suggestions in positive language.

Positive Consequences are much easier to accomplish than negative ones. 'I am becoming a permanent non-smoker' will produce a more successful result than 'I will give up smoking forever'. Every time.

Positively phrased Consequences are also more successful when they deal solely with you, rather than comparing you with anyone else. 'I am on the way to becoming a prominent fashion designer' is more likely to eventuate than 'I want to be more famous than Mandy'. 'I want to run the 100 metres in 11 seconds' is more influential than 'I want to be the fastest runner in my country'.

Make your Consequence specific, holistic and positive, and you are more likely to achieve it.

In the present Ambitions or Consequences expressed in the present tense are easier for your subconscious to take on board, and thus turn into reality.

This is why hypnotists say 'You are feeling sleepy', rather than 'You will fall asleep'.

There is something compelling about feeling you are part of NOW. Therefore, it is important to phrase and to imagine your Consequence as something that is happening NOW – not something that is going to happen, or will happen, but something that is in the process of happening at this very moment.

'I am feeling more calm and powerful with every page of this book.'

While it is not always practical to base your Consequence in the present, the process of achieving it should always be in the present – so that you are continually moving towards your Consequence.

Make your Consequence specific, holistic, positive and based in the present, and you are almost there.

Creating a powerful Consequence

Now we come to the part that transforms a Consequence you would normally express in words into something substantially more powerful (for most people).

When it comes to giving dimension to your Consequence, most of the self-help gurus urge you to write it down. 'Write it down on palm cards – place them in highly visible places, in your drawer, beside your bed, stuck to your bathroom mirror. Then refer to them often.'

Have you ever tried this? Did you feel like a bit of a failure when it didn't work? There is no need for you to feel this way, since this technique only works for some people. And it's easy to see why. Written words appeal to the logical, structured left side of the brain – and if you think you're going to produce big Consequences by using logic and linear thought processes (left-brain activities), you're going to be disappointed. It is virtually impossible to create integrated, holistic belief structures using reason and logic.

If we refer back to the Nine Mental Powers, we see that the subconscious is the most powerful way to influence your behaviour and thinking, and that once it takes on an idea, it immediately sets about trying to turn it into a reality. The Nine Mental Powers also tell us that the three ways to influence your subconscious are through repetition, emotion and imagination.

For simplicity's sake, I am not going to dwell on repetition other than to say that the more you mentally refer to your Consequence, the more you associate certain feelings and emotions with it, the more assured you are of realising it.

By definition, all Consequences are future-orientated. The only way to deal with the future is through your imagination (or mental images), a function of your right brain. Then you have *all* of your consciousness working towards fulfilling the Consequence you designate.

Speaking of images, have you noticed how everyone seems to be talking about visualisation these days? If you can visualise yourself achieving something, so the assurances go, you will eventually be able to achieve it. It is true that visualisation is one of the surest ways of influencing the subconscious. Problem is, most people can't visualise very well. At least not to the degree required to effect major change in their lives.

Each year thousands of corporations around the world dutifully prepare their 'vision statements' – carefully crafted expressions that supposedly summarise the future of the organisation in a few succinct words. In the main, these statements are masterpieces of fluff and verbiage. I've seen thousands of them. Even if we overlook the fact that most of them are poorly conceived – cliché-ridden and phrased more like legal documents than expressions of inspiration and ambition – they are still desperately limited in their vision. Why? They are usually just phrases of intent, and seldom possess any image-forming capabilities.

Can you imagine a vision without using (mental) images? Of course you can't.

A good storyteller uses words to create pictures in your mind. When I describe a coconut palm waving against a brilliant blue sky, with just a single white cloud drifting by, a picture forms in your mind. There's nothing you can do to prevent it. And if I add an overly tanned man in a red floral shirt, your mental picture becomes more complete. So, too, when I tell you about his scowling face, his straggly grey hair, plastic sandals and filthy feet. See? I can direct the content of your thoughts – from idyllic to disturbing in just three sentences – because I am providing the pictures.

But if I attempt to communicate this same scene to you by conveying basic information rather than pictures (as corporations tend to do in their vision statements), your mind remains unmoved. 'A man went to the beach.' Unless I provide the pictures, your subconscious has nothing to act on.

This same limitation exists when trying to design a Consequence for yourself. It requires more than words and data: it requires pictures.

I have made a discovery about visualisation: it is very rare for people to be able to visualise in any detail without some degree of assistance – especially when it comes to working on subtle personality shifts, or planning for their own achievements for life. If you were to ask them to *imagine* themselves doing specific things, or achieving specific things, they would do so easily. But ask them to *visualise* a bright, successful future for themselves and many would be left wondering, 'Where are the pictures?'.

So you will never need to ask this question in relation to *Calm for Life*, I will tell you how you can create the pictures that will describe the kind of Consequence that will work best for you.

The Consequence Montage

What follows may take a couple of hours to prepare. It may even cost a little to produce. But, because it will enable the most remarkable transformation in your thinking and capabilities, it is well worth the investment in time (and perhaps money).

We're going to create a success montage, or a wellness montage, or a calm montage, or a happiness montage. Whatever you call it, whatever its purpose, it will have the following attributes:

- specific, in the sense that it describes real, tangible, possibly even measurable results;

- holistic, in the sense that it does not seriously compromise your belief systems and values; and

- positive.

When completed, it will be a postcard-sized image of your Consequence which you can carry around with you, leave in your desk drawer, set on your bedside table, place on your bathroom mirror, and generally make part of your everyday life. The more this image is embedded in your subconscious, the more effectively it works.

You may think you have no skills in creating such images, but you will find that that is completely irrelevant to the few steps that lie ahead. The starting point of this montage is you. You will be the centre of it. Ideally, you would create most of this in your mirror – so you can see your own image as the central part. But most people (even vain ones) feel uncomfortable really exposing themselves in the mirror. So the means we will employ for this is a photograph.

Choosing the photograph   While any old photograph from your collection will do, the one we really want will satisfy a number of criteria.

For a start, it must be of you; your Consequence image *must* contain you at the centre. Next, this image should demonstrate (only to you) how you will feel when your Consequence is realised. This could involve special clothing – maybe you need to wear swimwear, or borrow a wedding dress, a smart suit or an Olympic medal for the occasion. But, most of all, it will show you in a particular emotional light. Almost surely, this light will be happy, well and calm, but in addition, your expression may be one of triumph, satisfaction, love, contentedness – your choice.

If you don't already have this photograph, buy two rolls of film and expose them all – just of you. Now you'll have between forty and eighty shots to choose from.

One of these shots will present you in the way that you believe is how you'll *feel* when your Consequence is realised. This is the photo we're going to work with in the creation of your Consequence Montage. (Don't be tempted to go for the most flattering photograph; choose the most compelling.)

It is possible that the Consequence you have in mind will be different to your photographic image. If your Consequence is to shed weight, for example, you may find that your existing image does not satisfy your requirements, and you might use an image that shows just your face . . . leaving the body to your imagination.

Modifying the photograph   Even with all those shots to choose from, and even if you find several of them show you in a flattering light, deep down you will not be completely satisfied with the result. 'They do not look like me.'

There is a reason for this lack of familiarity. You have only ever seen your face the mirror. That image was back-to-front. Reversed. A mirror image of the face that the rest of the world sees. So every time you see a photograph of yourself it is (in your view) back-to-front when compared with the image of yourself that is in your mind. Moreover, because the left and right sides of your face are quite different from one another, this disparity is emphasised.

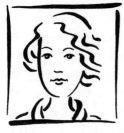

There is a simple way to overcome this. Have the photograph you have chosen printed back-to-front. This is a matter of flipping the negative before printing; any photo finisher can do it. Anyone else who sees this back-to-front photo may think there is something askew about it, but it will appear just right to you.

There's more. This flipped photograph may reveal something else about you. The human face is not symmetrical; one side is always slightly different from the other.

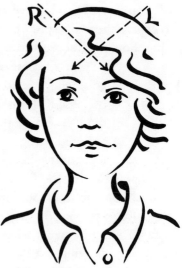

The left-hand side of your face is controlled by the right hemisphere of your brain (the creative, emotional, intuitive side), whereas the right-hand side of your face is controlled by your left brain (logical, structured).

Because of the different functions of each side of the brain, the result is a slightly different expression on either side of your face. Once again, this is something you wouldn't normally notice.

Because the right side of your face is being influenced by the logical, analytical side of your brain,

Public and private sides of the face

the expression it presents to the world is the one you'd like to present.

The left side of your face, though, tends to be a bit more revealing. As it is under the influence of the emotional side of your brain, it tends to be more honest about your inner thoughts and what you're really feeling. This is probably why it often appears a little more negative in its expression.

Fortunately, the left (private) side of your face is seldom as expressive as your right (public), so your innermost feelings are fairly well concealed.

You could go through life without ever consciously being aware of these variations in people's faces. Subconsciously, however, you would be quite aware of it. Subconsciously you know that, even though someone may be smiling nicely at you, the effect is insincere. Why? Because the insincerity is being expressed – subtly – in the left-hand side of their face. (If you want to test this, take the illustration above and hold it in front of a mirror. What you will see is a slightly different expression: more or less friendly; more or less sincere. Try it.)

Your instincts, your emotions, the opinions and feelings you have about yourself all emanate from the right brain. And are expressed on the left-hand side of your face. When you flip your photograph, you are exposing yourself to the right-hand side of your face. It is important, therefore, to review the photograph with this in mind. Off the top of your head, what does it communicate to you? Now that the photograph has been flipped, do you still look happy? Calm? Content? Don't think about it – what's it *feel* like? (A quick test is to hold the photo up to a mirror.)

If you have doubts, choose another photograph. Since you'll be living with it for quite a while, it's worth getting this right from the beginning.

Now take your completed photograph and mount it in the centre of a large piece of board.

Completing the image   Now you have an image that looks familiar (because it is similar to the image you see in the mirror) and desirable (because it shows you how you will eventually be) at the centre of your Consequence Montage. Whatever happens from hereon in, it is important that this image remains at the centre.

The completion of your Consequence Montage requires whatever additional elements will help you to visualise a powerful, successful, compelling picture of your future. These are images you can clip from magazines or picture books, or they can even be little sketches of your own. They could show a cheque, a *New York Times* bestseller list, a PhD, or a silhouette of two children and a spouse. They could even be certain words or shapes or phrases. This is an area where your own preferences and creativity come to the fore.

A book like this cannot be too prescriptive about what these elements should be, because they are meant to be personal; they will almost certainly mean things to you that others would not understand.

One interpretation of the Consequence Montage pictured over the page is that a woman, who is facing a very messy bankruptcy, has a desired Consequence of getting through this period to go on to live a calm and relaxed life by the sea, with her own house, her partner of several years and not a worry in the world. Of course, it would be constructed of photographs, magazine and newspaper clippings, and the like, not just drawings.

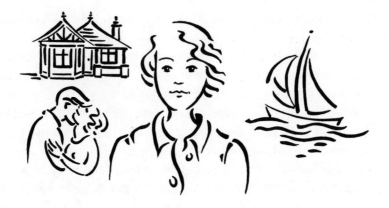

If you were facing a similar situation, your Consequence Montage would probably be completely different: not only in the elements it contained, but in the way they were portrayed. Whatever means most to you, whatever *feels* right – as opposed to whatever looks most artistic – is the way to go.

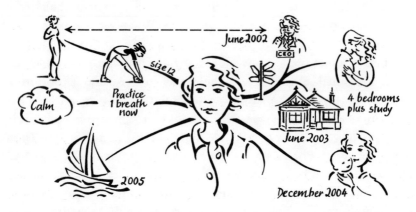

As this is the most personal expression you can imagine, you need not be limited to photographs. For example, the Consequence Montage above is embellished with words and instructions, which makes its goals more concrete. (You will note how each of the 'branches' leading away from the central figure deals with a different lifestyle attribute. Each of these branches could, in theory, have sub-branches – the 'house' branch, for example, could have layout or geographical detail attached to it.)

Your Consequence Montage can include dates, amounts, time

lines, ambitions, benchmarks – anything that makes it a meaningful map of your future. Be as extravagant in your design as you like. Get out your coloured pencils. Decorate the entire picture with colourful stars, or clouds, or seashells, if you think this would make it feel more powerful. There are no rules, no limitations.

At this stage, your Consequence Montage may be physically too large to carry about. So the next step involves going to a nearby photocopying service and getting the entire thing copied – in colour – and reduced to a postcard size, or any size you consider desirable. As this is the blueprint for your future, there's no point in skimping at this juncture. Order as many copies as you require. Have them laminated if you can; it will make your Consequence seem more fixed and substantial.

How to use it

Now that you have created your Consequence Montage, the next step is to put it to use.

You will need to refer to it often. A minimum of five times a day. Carry it with you. Place copies in all the places you visit regularly – particularly those places where you go alone and, ideally, are in a relaxed state. You might leave a copy on your beside table, your office desk, in your underwear drawer, on the bathroom mirror; I'm sure you'll think of other appropriate places.

The more you refer to it, and the more you associate certain feelings with it, the more integrated this image will become in your consciousness. Until one day . . . it happens. Your Consequence will be realised. And you may not even have noticed it. This transition is subtle and, for many people, goes unnoticed. Whether it takes place over 2 months or 10 years, it only becomes noticeable in retrospect. This is the beauty of fully integrated change. It happens unconsciously.

Sometimes, especially when there are benchmarks involved, there may be a surprise factor. For example, if you go back to your doctor and discover that you've made a full recovery, you may be surprised. As you might also be if your accountant phones you one day and says, 'You've got a million sitting in your cheque account, what are you going to do with it?'

In most instances, though, the change will not be noticeable until some time *after* it has taken place. What usually happens is that someone reminds you of what a stressed, depressed, unhappy or unsuccessful person you once considered yourself to be. I know this sounds a little magical: an extraordinary achievement or change in your life taking place without fanfare, without even being noticed, but that's how it happens for most people.

If your experience is like theirs, there will not be any break-through moment. There will be no surprise. And you may not even be aware of it at all, since what happens has already been integrated into your consciousness. Your subconscious will have made it so familiar, so 'real', that you will be convinced that it was always destined to happen. Someone may remind you that you read about this 'technique' in this book, but you will find it difficult to believe that this was the turning point.

'I was always going to do well as an architect. I've been training since high school and I put so much work into it.' (You forget that you once believed you were going to be a failure.)

'I was always going to take over as manager; it was just a matter of planning and time.' (You forget that, just 6 months ago, you were thinking about changing jobs.)

'I was always going to overcome breast cancer; I knew all along it would happen.' (You forget the extreme fear and doubt of earlier this year.)

'I was always going to be a world champion; I've been thinking about it since I was a child.' (You forget the sense of despair when you thought you were a sporting failure.)

'I was always going to be happy and contented, with a loving family. I was just going through a bad patch when I thought otherwise.'

You see the pattern? It happens this way in almost every case of real change – at least in most that I am aware of. The reason for this is that the path between integration and accomplishment starts incre-mentally as your subconscious begins to take your new belief on board, then continues exponentially as your subconscious sets about turning it into a reality. But at all stages the change will seem like the most natural, inevitable process you could imagine.

Perhaps this is to do with the growing familiarity of particular thought processes, and the establishment of more streamlined neural pathways. I am unsure. What I *am* sure about is that it happens: when your subconscious takes a Consequence on board and seamlessly transforms it into a new belief, you may not be aware of the process while it is happening, but it will happen.

The steps involved are:

- You are in a state that you want to change from

- You employ a technique designed to bring about change in precisely the way you want it

- When it happens, the change seems so natural and effortless, so much a part of you, that you find it difficult to contemplate that there was ever a possibility of it not happening.

Before you decided on a particular Consequence and adopted the techniques required to achieve it, you would have considered it a remote, if not impossible, prospect. But after formalising it in some way (such as in a Consequence Montage), and making it integral to your life using the success formula, your subconscious gradually convinces you it is not only realistic, but eminently achievable. Then, as far as your thoughts and beliefs are concerned, failure becomes an impossibility.

What could be easier than that?

You could be excused for thinking that working on the four elements we have covered – Consequence, Motivation, Belief and Focus – is all that's required to achieve miracles: to transform nervous wrecks into tranquil souls, lonely hearts into the loved and contented, everyday workers into wealthy successes, and even to eradicate incurable diseases. Some exceptional people will accomplish everything they desire using these four elements. But for most of us, it is next to impossible to accomplish the big things in life without additional assistance.

This is where *i* comes into the equation. And, when you use it, it increases the effectiveness of your Motivation, Belief and Focus by a substantial factor.

The power of *i*

For many years a specialisation of mine was the process of creativity. Not only did I operate in many facets of the arts (photography, art, music, fiction), but I also spent many years as a creative director and owner of advertising agencies. As a result, I have long had a professional interest in creativity – not just artistic creativity, but creative thinking in general: non-linear strategic planning for corporations, problem-solving techniques for business executives, stress-free creativity for people involved in the arts and marketing, and performance-enhancing creativity for sportspeople, investors, researchers, academics and so on.

In the process of doing this, my team identified a simple set of practices that had the potential to go way beyond professional applications. Thus began our explorations into the application of creativity in healing, depression, loneliness, stress relief, religion and business, as well as the arts.

The nub of this understanding is a quality or element which, for want of a better expression, we call i. 'i' stands for inspiration, intuition, imagination, I the personal pronoun, or any one of a number of different possibilities.

---

i and the Success Formula

To achieve anything significant in life – that is out of the ordinary when compared with your normal, everyday standards – you tend to adopt a certain procedure.

For the sake of convenience, I have formulated this as follows:

$$(M+B+F)^i = C$$

It works like this. First you make your Consequence real via an imaginative Consequence Montage. Next you have to match that with a proportionate measure of Motivation, Belief and Focus.

But to achieve an *extreme* Consequence (that is, one which seems extreme by your present standards), you need this extra ingredient, i – a stroke of inspiration, an out-of-the-ordinary creative solution.

But the more general application of i is one you can use every day of your life: as an effortless way of identifying the best course of action in any particular situation, or the most creative solution to a problem, or simply for your daily planning.

ì   is a gift from your subconscious and perhaps your unconscious mind.

ì   cannot be produced using reason, intellect, willpower or determination. In fact, the more you try to apply any of those forces, the further away from the solution you will be.

ì   *can only come from a state of calm.* While it can sometimes be accessed through stress or panic (via encroaching deadlines, fear of failure, or extreme threat), this is both unpredictable and inefficient.

ì   comes of its own accord. If you were focused and motivated, and had endless time and patience, this ì factor would probably make itself known to you. But you probably wouldn't recognise it when it did! Imagine being handed an inspired answer to a difficult problem, then struggling to find another solution because you didn't know you already had it.

The method I'm going to reveal is remarkably easy. It requires a little preparation and a few minutes of your time, but virtually no effort. What's more, even the slightest application of effort on your part will be counter-productive. The harder you try, the less will be the result. Doesn't that seem ideal?

(You might recall the second of the Calm Centre's Nine Mental Powers, the Power of Calm: in matters of the mind, the more mental effort you apply to any given situation, the less will be the result.)

The Calm Inspiration Cycle

Your subconscious is a remarkable 'place'. It is the repository of (or has direct access to) all you have ever experienced and known; all you have ever experienced and not consciously known about; and all you have ever experienced and thought you had forgotten. It has direct access to all your intuition and instincts. And to your wisdom. It knows more about you than your conscious mind does – infinitely more.

You can tap into the power of your subconscious by using the Calm Inspiration Cycle.

Before we explore this method in detail, there is one principle that needs to be established right from the outset:

The power of an idea bears no relationship to the time or effort taken to arrive at it.

Please remember that, because the Calm Inspiration Cycle makes ideas deceptively easy to access.

Many years ago I worked with a man in the business of producing commercial ideas for marketing organisations. As we were freelance we were paid by the idea rather than the hour, so we had a vested interest in working quickly. He was the fastest 'ideas' person I had ever worked with, and could arrive at innovative solutions almost as fast as a problem could be outlined.

Belief and trust

Belief and trust are sometimes interchangeable. You have probably experienced at least one example of how these can enhance the effectiveness of a simple mental procedure.

Have you ever gone to bed at night saying to yourself, 'I will wake at 6 a.m.'?

You repeat this to yourself a few times before falling asleep. Then, sure enough, next morning you wake just as the clock is passing 5.59 a.m.

'How did I do that?'

What's more, this technique works for you 100 percent of the time, with 100 percent accuracy, providing you do just one thing – trust that it will work.

If you doubt that it will work, it does not work. If you have doubts, you wake at 4.43 a.m., again at 4.59, again at 5.27, again at 5.35, then you sleep through to your usual waking time of 8.30.

If you trust in your own instincts, this wake-up technique will work for you 100 percent of the time, with 100 percent effectiveness.

Initially, we thought it might be unprofessional to rely on these flashes of inspiration, but after a few months we learned to have faith in his instincts. Soon I learned to trust my own in a similar way.

What came out of that relationship was a simple, problem-solving or idea-producing formula. If you use this formula as I am going to explain it, you will come up with the most inspired solution you are humanly capable of – at that particular moment. Better still, you will do this 100 percent of the time.

In case you missed that fact, let me reiterate:

> *This formula will provide the most inspired*
> *solution you are humanly capable of – at that*
> *particular moment – 100 percent of the time.*

At the core of this procedure are three simple steps. They will seem simple. Take care not to confuse simplicity with ineffectiveness, because if you trust in them they will work for you in an inspired fashion.

The three stages are:

- Start at the end
- Go to the centre
- Accept the answer

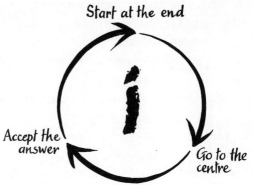

Start at the end In another life, when I was involved in strategic planning for businesses, I discovered something about people who work in the corporate sector: most of them don't know how to plan. At first I thought this was a shortcoming peculiar to businesses, then it became obvious that most people use the same limited approach.

When you're planning an event in the future, where do you start?

If you're hoping to work your way through a difficult problem, where do you start?

If you're seeking a creative answer to a perplexing question, where do you start?

Most people start in exactly the same place: the beginning.

Earlier, when we compared reductionism and holism (pages 71–4), we saw the reason for this. As human beings we've been trained to address mental activity in a certain way: start at the beginning and work your way through. Linear, logical, methodical. But not very smart.

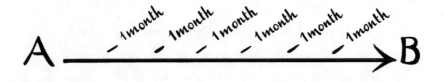

This linear approach is meant to work in a predictable way. Your starting point is now. Today. This moment (A in the diagram above). Reality. You say to yourself, 'Here I am today: lonely, out of work, having difficulty paying the rent. In 6 months, I'd love to be in a fun job where I could be well paid and meet interesting people. What do I do next?' Then you start planning or thinking it through. One logical step after the other – away from the reality of now, and all the things you know to be true – off towards some vague situation in the future (B in the diagram).

This kind of approach is more suited to calculation than creativity. It takes a structured, analytical, logical (or left-brain) approach to an issue that defies linear thinking: thinking about the future. In the overwhelming majority of cases, it doesn't work. You simply can't have a vision of the future using your left brain. That's not how the mind works.

The future can only exist in the imagination, which is a function of the right brain. For this reason, any attempt at planning or trying to shape the future in your mind must use *right-brain* methods. The method that does this most effectively is the reverse of the approach that most people use.

In other words, you start at the *end* (B). You begin with a situation of fantasy or a figment of your imagination: 'Here I am on 30 June,

B

– 1 month

– 1 month

– 1 month

– 1 month

– 1 month

– 1 month

↓

A

6 months from now. I'm working in a wonderful restaurant – the tips are great – with a really great team of people. I'm meeting new people every night. It's exciting.'

Then, using your imagination, you start working backwards to 'now' (A). And at various intervals along the way, you stop and ask yourself, 'What did I do to get here?'

It works infinitely better than the other way. And it works because it relies on the part of you that deals with abstract concepts like the future – the creative, picture-forming, *right* side of your brain. It works because it can tap into your subconscious and unconscious mind as well as your conscious. And it is a far more holistic way to plan.

You start at the end and work back.

What's more, you do it in your mind: you imagine what you'd look like after you have achieved what you set out to achieve. Take note of what you'd see when you're in this position, and the sounds you'd hear. Then imagine what it would *feel* like once you'd achieved this objective you have in mind. Your starting point is where you want to end up.

Before you begin this solution-finding process, you will have in mind a clear idea of what you want to achieve. In effect, this is a brief to yourself. A well-formulated Consequence.

Go to the centre   The next stage in this process is to open your mind to the answer.

As we have discovered, you cannot force yourself to come up with an inspired answer, and you cannot bring about innovative or creative insights by applying intellect or thinking hard. The big answers, the breakthrough answers, come from the most relaxed states.

So the second stage in this process is going to your centre – the place you *perceive* as your centre. Your calm centre. Deep Calm. You can use any of the techniques in Step 3 (pages 145–70) to do this.

The most important consideration is that, during this process, you try to think about your problem. You occupy your consciousness with any of the methods we covered in Step 3, and you try not to think about what you hope to achieve – you simply enjoy the exercise.

Accept the answer Now we come to the most challenging stage of this process.

It is challenging because the answers are presented by your subconscious. Often, your *conscious* mind doesn't like to listen to these types of answers. Often, your conscious mind argues that whatever cannot be worked out by logic, reason and hard mental effort (that is, conscious effort), cannot possibly be of use.

But this is where your conscious mind misleads you. And since your conscious mind has not served you so handsomely to date – it hasn't helped you in becoming calm at will, increasing your happiness, enhancing your physical and mental health, or accomplishing your more challenging objectives – you may rightfully assume that it should not be heeded on this occasion.

Therefore the challenge in this particular step is to accept whatever answers come to mind – *without analysis*. This is the difficult part. All your life you've operated the same way: when you have a thought or idea, you immediately evaluate it according to a range of biases and experiences – then adopt it, develop it further or discard it, according to this assessment.

I call this process 'self-editing'. It happens to all people to a greater or lesser degree, and becomes more pronounced as you get older. It eventuates after you've tried and discarded a particular approach to a set of circumstances at some stage of your life. The next time a similar set of circumstances arises, you say, 'No, that approach doesn't work' or 'I can't do that'. These are self-limiting generalisations. Left unchecked, they progressively limit your capacity to appreciate new experiences and to be open to new ways of thinking.

Your conscious mind specialises in self-editing. It compares all present experiences, and all imaginary (future) experiences with what has gone before, then it starts to edit: 'I've never been able to do that'; 'My sister tried that, it didn't work for her'; 'No-one I know has ever succeeded using that approach'; 'People can't relate to that sort of thing'.

And the more you do this, the fewer tastes, experiences,

personalities and behaviours you can accept. This is very limiting. And very unnecessary.

All throughout your day, your subconscious communicates with you. It does this through feelings, impressions, hunches and impulses. When these come along, you have a choice: heed them or reject them.

The tendency of your conscious mind is to reject them. After all, they're 'just feelings'. And, by heeding them, you run the risk of being assessed as emotional, impulsive or arcane. But, as we've examined in an earlier chapter, *all* creativity and inspiration comes from your subconscious or unconscious. All of it. This means that all the great ideas you have had, and will have in the future, stem from this one place.

When you know what you want to achieve (Start at the end), then go to a state of deep relaxation (Go to the centre), your subconscious will present you with a range of suggestions.

You must be open to these suggestions. Moreover, you must accept whatever answers come to mind – *without analysis*. To do this, you'll need to find a quiet place in your home, office, garden or wherever.

Do not speak to anyone! You do not want to start turning your subtle thoughts (which will be flowing by this stage, although you may be unaware of them) into words – shifting them from your subconscious into your conscious mind; shifting them from right-brain feelings into left-brain words. There is one other step that must be accomplished first – and this requires two accessories.

The first is a large pad, preferably larger than a writing pad. *And it must be unlined.* Lined paper is designed to enforce conformity and encourage linear thinking – the last things we require here. (As one prominent man in advertising once encouraged his colleagues: 'If they give you lined paper, write sideways'.)

The second accessory is a thick-leaded pencil, or a thick-tipped felt pen.

It's important to choose a thick point so that you will be inclined to use it in broad strokes. Detail is not only unnecessary at this stage, it is undesirable.

The moment you emerge from Deep Calm, go to the quiet place you've chosen, pick up your pencil and write whatever comes to mind on your large pad. Don't think about it. Just start writing, drawing, making marks or whatever – do some-thing. As long as you don't try to overlay any intelligent perspective on this, you will intuitively choose the right marks or words because your subconscious will be directing you.

Although you may not know it yet, this is *i*. Or at least the begin-ning of *i*.

There will be times when you will have no idea of any specific answer. This is a perfectly acceptable result. Accept it. Be thankful for it.

How can this be? What sort of answer is no answer at all?

Say you were searching for guidance on how to deal with a health issue. In this situation, a clearly articulated answer regarding your ail-ment or its remedy may not be all that meaningful. Or that helpful. You might be far better served simply knowing *intuitively* what to do, what action to take. Here, feelings and intuition can be considerably more useful than conscious revelations.

Most times, though, what you write will be a completely formu-lated idea that sits in the forefront of your consciousness.

Symbol vs thought

Why is it that, sometimes, you will have a mysterious, symbolic, per-haps difficult-to-understand feeling, and at other times you will have a beautiful, fully formed thought? This is usually determined by the specific state of Deep Calm you experienced.

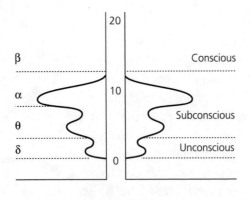

Thought states

If your state showed elevated alpha-relaxed and theta-open brainwave frequencies (as is most common in meditative states), the answers you receive will tend to be fully formed thoughts.

Generally, the alpha-relaxed frequencies provide the bridge between your conscious and subconscious (and unconscious); if these alpha frequencies are depressed or absent, this communication has to work in different ways.

This is why if your state shows elevated theta-open brainwave frequencies with substantially reduced alpha-relaxed frequencies, as in the graph below, the answers provided by your subconscious will not be so clear-cut – at least not as far as your conscious mind is concerned. All you will have is a *feeling*, a hunch, or a few scattered words, pictures, or symbols.

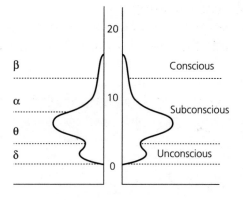

Symbol/feeling states

Whichever way they arrive, these are gifts from your subconscious. Accept them. Be grateful for them. Consciously note that it was your subconscious which helped you to find them. Then, the next time you do this exercise it will work even more efficiently for you.

You've accepted your answers. You are aware of no more subconscious inspirations that should be jotted down on your pad. Now, walk away. Give the task no more thought for a few minutes – perhaps until after you've had a cup of tea, or read your emails.

Interpretation

Now we come to the interpretation phase. If your answers were not fully formed ideas, it is time to turn whatever you have drawn on your pad into concrete answers or suggestions.

This is a simple left-brain process. You look at the words and/or symbols and ask, 'What does this mean to me? What was my subconscious/unconscious telling me?'

Sometimes there will be no clear-cut answer to this question. Other times it will be blindingly obvious, in which case you will need to continue this process no further.

But what if you can't fathom what the symbols mean? What if, after evaluating the answers you've accepted, you were to say, 'This is not right for me because it overlooks one important piece of information I'd forgotten about'?

The procedure to follow is best explained by the following case study. It's the story of someone I once worked with.

The 'need' in this story may not seem all that great to you, but for the woman concerned, it dominated her life. The story involves a highly competent lawyer we'll call Kate. She did not see herself as a highly competent lawyer; all she could see was someone who was overweight, who was inclined to wheeze after modest exertion, and who was 'forced' to dress in black so her weight would be less noticeable. When her doctor informed her that her blood pressure was high, and that she must lose weight to get it back to normal, she was distressed. Dieting had never worked for her before. What could she possibly do?

First, **Start at the end.**

Kate knew what she wanted to achieve. The problem was that 'losing weight' was hardly a positive Consequence. And 'lowering my blood pressure' was hardly imaginative, or specific.

So she decided to turn both of those objectives into a positive, optimistic, *visual* Consequence – one she could easily imagine. So instead of concentrating on blood pressure or diet, she formed a mental picture of herself as she would like to be: healthy, happy, full of energy and in a bright-coloured size 12 dress. The dress was an important visual benchmark in this process.

In Kate's mind she *was* healthy, happy, full of energy and wearing a size 12 dress. She spent a couple of minutes just luxuriating in that feeling.

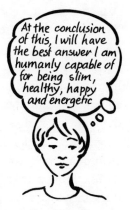

Then, before moving on to the next step, we suggested a brief for her:

'At the conclusion of this, I will have the best answer I am humanly capable of for being slim, healthy, happy and energetic. What steps did I take to get here?'

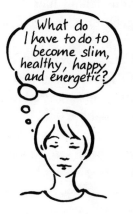

After a few minutes of this, Kate did not feel those words were strong enough for her. So, to add a little more impetus to this issue, we turned the words into a question: 'What do I have to do to become slim, healthy, happy and energetic?'

(You may find one way works better than the other for you. Whichever *feels* more natural is the one to go with.)

Let's continue with Kate's story.

Next, **Go to the centre**. As she had been practising the Breath of Calm (page 153) each evening when she came home, she was now ready to make this work for her – by using it to go to her calm centre. She spent 20–30 minutes sitting quietly, concentrating on the sound of her breathing and soon she was enjoying the state of Deep Calm. While in this state, *she gave no thought at all to the Consequence she had planned*.

At the conclusion of this, she went straight to a quiet place in her garden to **Accept the answer**. On this occasion, she did not have a complete answer sitting in the forefront of her consciousness. So, using a large pad and thick-leaded pencil, the first mark she made on the page was a picture of the rising sun. She had no idea if it meant anything or not, she just felt like drawing it. Next, she wrote down the word 'vegetable'. This made sense. And it led to a predictable list of other words: 'salad', 'wholefood', 'celery', 'fibre'.

On a roll now, she started to get carried away with her writing and drawing – it didn't matter what it meant, she was enjoying the exercise.

A picture of an apple. She wrote a few words off the top of her head. 'Noon.' 'Mark.' These were not making sense to her. She wondered if she was doing it right. 'Diary.' What could these words mean?

As these words, pictures, symbols and feelings were communications from her subconscious, Kate noted and was grateful for this fact. Then, after a few minutes' break, it was time to analyse them: reviewing them to see if they satisfied her needs, testing them against her pre-conceptions, seeing if they could be improved upon – and, crucially, examining them to see if they had meanings she might have missed.

She looked at the picture of the rising sun and wondered, 'What does this mean to me? What is my subconscious telling me?' She *thought* it might mean something like, 'I should get up earlier each day and exercise'.

Then she looked at the word 'vegetable'. There was no mystery here. Primarily, this reminded her that her diet featured too many meat dishes – and that the answer was to substitute more vegetables. (This also explained 'salad', 'wholefood', 'celery' and 'fibre'.)

The picture of the apple could have been a simple continuation of that thought. Or maybe not. Could an apple have some other meaning? Of course! She'd read about a way of eating where before noon you ate only fruit. Supposedly it helped you to become trim and healthy in a very short period. That probably explained the word 'noon' as well.

She had no idea what the word 'mark' meant. Did it mean bench-mark? Marking time? Exam marks? She could think of nothing. (Sometimes there will be no clear-cut answer to a particular word or symbol.) Pass on to the next.

The final word on her page was 'diary'. Perhaps if she were to change her diet to include more vegetables, and eat only fruit before noon each day, and rise an hour earlier to exercise each day, it would be a good idea to keep a diary of these activities to plot the progress of her new state of health and vitality.

That was all for the moment. Later in the day, as she thought about these issues, the idea of that new way of eating excited her. She could see how such a dietary regime could be linked to that mental picture of herself in a bright-coloured size 12 dress. Yes, she would definitely adopt that way of eating. Immediately.

What about that picture of the rising sun? Unfortunately, rising an hour earlier each day to exercise did not appeal in the least. Maybe it meant something else. Maybe she'd have to force herself to overcome that dislike of exercise. It made sense.

And, although she was not dwelling on this during the day, the word 'mark' didn't mean anything in particular to her. She had been warned that this was quite common and was nothing to lose sleep over.

At 7.30 that evening, she called from her car. Excited. She knew what 'mark' meant and it was going to make all the difference to her life. Some 6 months earlier she had been introduced to the brother of a friend. His name was Mark. Not only was he cute, but he was also a fitness trainer. At the time she'd thought the notion of a personal trainer was the height of self-indulgence. But now it made sense! She had already called him and was about to commence an early-morning training program with him on Monday.

You know how things turned out for Kate?

Precisely. She's healthy, happy, full of life, and wearing a size 12 dress. She still wears black, though. (Mark prefers dark colours on her.)

You might say this sounds obvious. Maybe it does. But it wasn't obvious to Kate, who'd been wrestling with this issue for years. Of course she now 'knows' that it was Mark who provided the solution, not anything as intangible as her subconscious.

But she still uses the above technique for *all* of her major work issues: Start at the end; Go to the centre; Accept the answer.

These three steps form the core of a larger formula, the complete Calm Inspiration Cycle.

The complete Calm Inspiration Cycle

Sometimes the issues that confront you require major, life-changing decisions. On such occasions, the formula we have just explored may require an additional measure of inspiration. This is provided by the complete Calm Inspiration Cycle.

Inspiration, creativity, *i* – call it what you will – is the product of your subconscious mind. No amount of intellect or mental effort can produce it.

Given enough preparation and a relaxed atmosphere, inspiration may come of its own accord. If you sit around waiting long enough, something will usually arise. Some of us don't live that long, though.

If you want creativity or inspiration to happen on *your* terms, in the time frame that *you* designate, then you will need a different approach. And, if you want it to happen as a disciplined response to a brief that you outline, it must follow a certain procedure. The complete Calm Inspiration Cycle is that procedure.

While there are seven steps involved, this is not a complicated procedure. Indeed, it is probably the way you already address most of your *successful* problem-solving situations.

1.   Preparation
2.   *Start at the end*
3.   *Go to the centre*
4.   *Accept the answer*
5.   Conscious evaluation
6.   Unconscious evaluation
7.   Integration

The complete Calm Inspiration Cycle is like many skills in life – skiing, driving a car, swinging a golf club, playing the guitar. In the early stages you employ a number of well-defined steps: 'Your left hand goes here, first finger on this string, second finger on this one; rest the guitar on your left thigh; your right hand . . .', and so on.

However, after you have done this a few times, many of these steps integrate. They become second nature. When you reach that stage – to continue the guitar-playing analogy – you automatically adopt the correct posture and place your hands in the desired position without thinking. Then it simply becomes a matter of looking at a chord chart, checking your finger positions, and playing. Later, after you have practised this way for some time, you no longer have to check your finger positions: you just look at the chord chart and play.

After you have used the complete Calm Inspiration Cycle a few times, you will find yourself refining it to the three central steps (2, 3, 4) for most everyday situations.

Please remember, though, that in situations of great need — such as in a crisis or when facing serious illness — you need to follow all steps in detail. No matter how many times you have used this procedure, go back to basics and follow all the steps.

1. Preparation   This is the conscious effort part, the homework part. It is entirely left-brain in its operation, and is the step people usually feel most at home with. You perform this in a beta-intense state, using all your conscious faculties.

Essentially, this is the data-gathering part. You study your topic. You research, prepare, compare, calculate, evaluate, explore, assess. This part of the equation might take half an hour, or it might take 5 years. It's no different from any other undertaking in life; you must do your preparatory work first.

Let's use Kate's example again. (I will fantasise a little here, because I don't know the inner workings of her mind.) She's determined to become more fit and healthy. But how?

Just look at some of the things she might do as she prepares to create the new Kate:

- read every health and fitness magazine on the market

- speak to a dietician

- have a medical check-up

- pore over the fashion magazines, wondering what she might wear when she gets into shape

- visit the local gym to check out exercise programs

- observe every person in the street where she works, taking note of their shape and their demeanour

- go to the library to read up on body shape and dietary issues.

She could have accomplished all of this in a matter of hours. In Kate's case, it took a couple of months. By then, she had a mind full of information and data, but every time she sat down to plan her transformation program, she came to the same tired old conclusion: she had tried it before, it didn't work, so what was the point in trying it again?

At the conclusion of a process like this you may have lucked upon the answer. Usually, though, you will have nothing more than the resources to formulate a brief for yourself. In Kate's case, this brief worked best in question form: 'What do I have to do to become slim, healthy, happy and energetic?'

And that was it. She had consciously researched, studied, explored, calculated and gathered data, then formulated a brief for herself. (If you ever have difficulty formulating a brief for yourself, simply use the core three steps – Start at the end, Go to the centre, Accept the answer. At the conclusion of this process you should have the ideal set of words.)

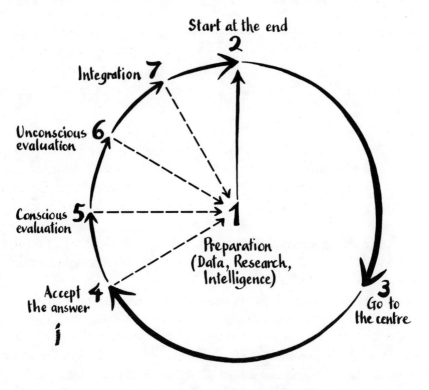

The complete Calm Inspiration Cycle

2. Start at the end At the conclusion of the Preparation stage, you will have a brief to yourself. If you take this brief and turn it into a Consequence that is as real as your imagination is capable of, you know exactly where you want to be at the completion of this cycle. This is your starting point: you start where you want to end up.

Kate started with: 'At the conclusion of this, I will have the best answer I am humanly capable of for being slim, healthy, happy and energetic'. She imagined how she'd look after she'd achieved this objective: fit, healthy, energetic, breezing around in a bright-coloured size 12 dress. (Note that she did not concentrate on the area that was hardest to become motivated about – lowering her blood pressure.)

3. Go to the centre You have decided on where you want to end up – your Consequence. Now it's time to take it easy. Just relax.

Using one of the Step 3 techniques (pages 145–70), allow yourself to go to your calm centre. Do not think about your brief to yourself, or the answers you require. Concentrate only on the relaxation method you have chosen, until you reach a state of Deep Calm.

4. Accept the answer After visiting your calm centre for 20–30 minutes, maybe longer, your subconscious will provide you with a range of suggestions – words, pictures, symbols, feelings or whatever. Some of these will be clear, some not so clear. Write them all down, in broad strokes, on a large pad, with a thick-leaded pencil.

These are gifts from your subconscious. Accept them. Be grateful for them. Do that, and the next time you perform this process it will work even more effectively for you.

Sometimes you will immediately see the answer, other times it may takes hours or even days. Other times, you will immediately know that the answer is not what you're looking for – in which case, you simply repeat the process and return to the Preparation stage.

5. Conscious evaluation You have your answers. Now for the easy part: you can be as critical as you like of those answers – a simple, left-brain process. 'What does this mean to me? What is my subconscious telling me?'

In Kate's case, would it be practical to adopt a fruit-only diet before noon? Is that a sensible diet? How long before the novelty wears off? Adding more vegetables to her diet sounds fine, but meat is so much easier to cook. Would that help lower her blood pressure?

Now you (and Kate) come to the first crossroads. You are faced with one of two possibilities:

(i) Accept the answers. In the event that you do, continue the complete Calm Inspiration Cycle with the next step, unconscious evaluation.

(ii) Reject the answers because they are impractical or inappropriate at this moment. In this case, you move straight back to the first step, Preparation, which means reviewing the data, gathering more if necessary, doing more research, reading more magazines, visiting the library . . . until such time as you feel that you have sufficient information to restart the process with a refined brief to yourself.

For example, Kate might change her brief to: 'At the conclusion of this, I will have the best answer I am humanly capable of to *gradually becoming a healthy, happy and energetic size 12*'.

6. Unconscious evaluation Assuming you have consciously examined your answer and see no substantial problems with it, it is now time to put it to your unconscious, or subconscious, to see if it is really acceptable to you at the deepest levels. This is the only way to ensure that your answers, or your new way of thinking, can work harmoniously and holistically with you.

This process can be fun, imaginative and should only take a few minutes. If you like, you can save it for the next time you're performing one of the Step 3 exercises.

Go somewhere where you will not be disturbed for 10 minutes, but choose somewhere different from where you went during stages 4 and 5 – this separation of locations is important. Sit quietly for a minute or so, listening to the sound of your breathing. When you feel deeply relaxed, imagine yourself having achieved your Consequence.

When you feel comfortable with that image, imagine yourself adopting the measures your subconscious has suggested to you. Are you happier, more content? Do you *feel* that they are working for you?

In Kate's case, she imagined herself adopting the fruit-only diet before noon; although she had doubts about the wisdom of the diet, it felt good to her. Then she imagined herself waking an hour earlier some days to exercise with her personal trainer, Mark. Surprise of surprises, she did not feel self-conscious but actually felt good about it.

7. Integration So your answer has passed the Conscious evaluation as well as the Unconscious evaluation. Now it's time to apply the answer, to integrate it.

The process of Integration is simply putting into effect the answers your subconscious has provided. And to do that, we have a powerful formula:

$$(M+B+F)^i = C$$

That is all there is to the Calm Inspiration Cycle. Simple, isn't it?

In each instance, the Calm Inspiration Cycle will provide the most inspired solution you are humanly capable of – at that particular moment. It always works, and it always works effectively, as long as you put your trust in it (just as when you tell yourself you're going to wake at a certain time, and trust in the process, you always wake on the dot). The words to note here are 'at that particular moment'. You may be able to improve on the result by varying your Preparation stage and modifying your brief. The only way of knowing whether there is a better way or not is to apply the Conscious evaluation and Unconscious evaluation steps.

How long does this take?

The steps outlined above need not be time-consuming. As with any new skill, you spend longer at it when you are learning the process than when it's familiar to you.

I use variations on this technique almost every day of my life. I use it to do all my business planning in a very short time. Most days I plan a whole day's work in 40 minutes – then spend the rest of the day following the suggestions made by my subconscious.

In the beginning, the time required for the complete Calm Inspiration Cycle is approximately as follows:

1. Preparation . . . . as long as it takes

2. *Start at the end* . . . . 5 minutes

3. *Go to the centre* . . . . 20–45 minutes

4. *Accept the answer* . . . . 5–15 minutes

5. Conscious evaluation . . . . 5–15 minutes

6. Unconscious evaluation . . 10–15 minutes

7. Integration . . . . ongoing

After you have performed this a few times, you will probably shorten the process so that you knowingly perform only steps 2, 3 and 4 – although you will generally perform the other steps unconsciously. After you have become familiar with those three steps, and have used them successfully a number of times, you will find that even they can be abbreviated. And this abbreviation continues until you get to the stage where the whole process of inspiration becomes one easy, fluid process that you can bring into play at any time.

Interpreting the answer

Most people find that their subconscious communicates in a very straightforward way: a simple idea springs to mind and they say, 'That's it!'

Others find that the subconscious communicates with hints and suggestions rather than concrete ideas. Or intuition and feelings, hunches, if you like. Or symbols and images – sometimes very complete images. If this is your experience, learn how to record these images *without turning them into words*.

What is important is that you remain open to suggestion after completing stages 1–4, then take note of how your subconscious likes to communicate. We're all different. And, as we saw on pages 220–1, the subconscious communicates differently depending on the state of Deep Calm we experience.

Finally, learn to pay attention to your hunches and intuition in these circumstances. If you really *feel* something is the right answer, then chances are it will be the right answer for you. How often have you experienced this: you think of an answer, review it, say to yourself, 'There must be more to it than that', then spend days working through the alternatives – only to return to your first answer after all?

Intuition is one of your most powerful resources. You've been taught to ignore this force, and perhaps even to discredit it – usually in favour of knowledge. Your instincts tell you that a certain course of action is the one you should pursue, and your head tells you something else. You have been educated to believe that what your head tells you is the way to go.

Much of the time, this is a fallacy. As we have explored throughout this book, the fact that you see something, or 'know' something, does not mean it is so. Yet, isn't your intuition a manifestation of your subconscious *knowledge*? Intuition is not invention; it is simply applying knowledge that you cannot consciously access. And you can't consciously access it because you've either forgotten it, or were unaware that you'd witnessed it. This latter occurrence applies to 99 percent of the information that's around you – you are not consciously aware of it, but it's all being recorded by your subconscious.

There is an old Buddhist saying that is usually translated along the lines of: 'When the student is ready, the master will appear'. That means, when you start looking for the answer, the answer will turn up.

You see this in all aspects of life.

When I'm writing my books and preparing an outline, I know that within months of starting to write, people will contact me out of the blue with information that I need. Not so long ago, when I was writing *Calm at Work*, a European colleague mentioned a book called *The Rebirth of Nature* by Rupert Sheldrake. I searched everywhere for it, with no success. Then, within 24 hours of initiating the search, I found a copy that had been abandoned in the first-class lounge at Changi Airport in Singapore.

Coincidence? How about this, then?

While I was researching this book, a diver told me about his experience of brainwave entrainment in the presence of dolphins and whales. Just as I was preparing to head off to the university library in search of scientific confirmation of this phenomenon, I received an email from Dr Peter Beamish (author of *Dancing With Whales*), who was not only an expert on whales and their communications, but also recognised similarities between his work and what my other books had been suggesting. Until that email, I had never heard of him.

In a section in Chapter 8, I was writing the words, 'Asking an author about relationships is a little like asking a prisoner about life on the other side . . .'(see page 306), when my fax machine spilled out a message. It was from a prison psychologist wanting to make contact about *Calm at Work*.

I have dozens of such examples that relate specifically to the writing and research of my books. Almost every author and scriptwriter I know has had a similar experience: they decide to write a story about giant monkeys, runaway toy trains, skiing nuns or whatever, and by the time they've developed the project they hear of someone working in parallel – usually someone on the other side of the world with no connection with them whatsoever.

You may call this coincidence, but it is more accurately known as synchronicity, where two people have the same thought, or decide to communicate, at the same instance.

You have probably experienced synchronicity with people close to you – both of you will raise the same obscure topic at the same instant; he or she will answer your question before you ask it; you know exactly what the next question he or she is going to ask you will be. Synchronicity. It is such a widespread experience (for people who are open to it) that you could hardly call it a phenomenon. However, in the world of science, it is considered a phenomenon and, as a result, there are millions being spent trying to discover why people have this experience.

There is a growing number of biologists, physicists and cosmologists who are fascinated by the potential of 'coincidences'. One of these, Rupert Sheldrake, has developed a Morphic Field Theory, which explains the inter-connectedness of consciousness in nature through bioenergetic fields. Maybe it is a bioenergetic field that helps you to find the answers you are looking for. Maybe it's coincidence. Maybe it's the collective consciousness that Jung wrote about. Maybe it's alien messengers. Maybe it is, as I've been saying all along, a communication from your subconscious. It doesn't really matter; all that matters is that you find the answers you are looking for – and the fact that you are looking, and are open to what you may receive, means they will appear.

Some time back I wrote a book called *The Little Book of Calm*. Basically, it was a series of suggestions that could help trigger a calm state in individuals. Knowing that readers would take whatever meaning they chose from these words – if they were invited to do so – rather than just accepting them at face value, I urged them to 'let this book fall open – let your intuition guide you – and you will see the most effective way for you to find calm *at that particular moment*'.

I have a hard disk full of emails from readers who make astonishing discoveries for themselves that extend way beyond the literal interpretation of my words. The reason they found what they were looking for has little to do with the brilliance of my words; because they were searching for an answer, and were open to it, an answer appeared.

I will share one more story with you before I leave you to your own devices in your search for the answers you require.

In 1998 I spoke at a function called 'Alternatives' in St James's, a wonderful Christopher Wren-designed church in London's Piccadilly. As I looked out into the audience, humbled by the history of the place and by the luminaries who had lectured from this same spot before me, I noticed a dishevelled-looking woman with red-dened eyes sitting at the back. For the following hour, I kept noticing this one face in the audience. At the conclusion of the event, there was that same face at the end of the book-signing line.

'I picked up your book in a bookshop,' she said, opening a battered copy of *The Little Book of Calm*. 'I opened it at this page.'

The heading at the top of the page said: 'Recognise addiction'. It was a simple thought about the addictive nature of caffeine and how it could fool you into believing it was relaxing when, in fact, it was stimulating.

'I've been in detox since the day after I read that.'

I still communicate with this woman from time to time. She insists to this day that what she read on the page of that book was quite specific to her need. She found what she needed, because she was open to the answer.

Life is as simple as that.

You will discover this for yourself when you search, and are open to the answer. Learn to trust your intuition. The more open you are, the surer you are of finding a solution. This is the power of **i**.

Life design

In this chapter, you have discovered how to design your Consequence and to present it in its most compelling form, so it will stimulate the required levels of motivation, belief and focus to achieve it.

There will come times, though, when your decisions and actions have life-long implications: in the areas of goal-setting, career, relationships, health and so on. At these times, you may need to take a broader approach to formulating your Consequence.

The starting point for this is the issue of your life itself. What is your purpose in life? Why are you here? How do you intend to give *your* life consequence?

Those whose lives are defined by a sense of purpose derive more satisfaction and suffer fewer insecurities than those whose lives lack purpose.

Does your life have purpose? If not, the following technique will help you determine your purpose in life.

When I was in high school, we had a program called the Adventure Course. Several teams would be given a cross-country course, then it became a race to see who could get to a designated point first. The first time I led a team, our objective was to reach the peak of a small mountain at the rear of our school grounds. There was one major peak and two smaller, almost like three separate mountains.

It was not a difficult slope. The course we chose, however, was directly through a lantana thicket, which meant hacking through prickly shrub with machetes. After half a day of scratches, leeches and blisters, we emerged from the thicket to discover we were only a third of the way up the slope. The remaining two-thirds were easier. If we hurried, we would be able to make the peak in a few more hours. We made it in reasonably good time.

The only problem was, when we finally made it, we discovered it was the wrong peak.

I often think back on that event as being a powerful metaphor for life's efforts. What if, after you've invested all your effort in a certain path, you find you've climbed the wrong mountain?

So that you can avoid this frustration, I'm going to introduce you to a very simple exercise. It's called the Centenarian Test. The purpose of this test is to identify the fundamental issues that you believe are most important to your life. This should be an easy question to answer. *Shouldn't it?*

Unfortunately not. While I was writing *Calm at Work* my researchers conducted a number of surveys into people's attitudes towards their work. Frequently, the question that caused most perplexity was 'Why do you go to work?' Naturally, everyone had an immediate answer. But when they sat down and thought about it, in very few cases did that answer really mean a lot to them. Don't you find this surprising in a world that is so devoted to personal development, goal-setting, benchmarking and job enrichment? If people have trouble with a simple question like 'Why do you go to work?', imagine how they baulked at the next question: 'What is most important in your life?'

Most people go through life without ever really pausing and exploring what is fundamental to their needs in life. The Centenarian Test will show you how to do just that. More importantly, it will help you dispense with the glib answers – the ones you provide for yourself, as much as for other people.

For such a simple test, it can be extraordinarily revealing. And, usually, the answers will get more revealing each time you do it. I'll give you an example. If you ask most people 'What is most important in your life?' you'll get an answer that covers some vague ideal like 'happiness'. Whenever I hear this I become suspicious. Suspicious? Surely everyone wants to be happy . . .

I do not believe this. An Oxford psychologist, Robert Holden (author of *Happiness Now* and creator of the Happiness Project), has devoted much of his professional life to spreading happiness: teaching people how they can become happy with a minimal investment of time and effort. Considering the profound nature of this possibility, I added the question 'What is most important in your life?' to a small survey we were conducting among successful businesspeople.

Guess what? Happiness was not rated very highly as a goal. In the instances where it *was*, the person in question was invariably one we could categorise as 'unhappy'. So unhappy people saw happiness as one of the most important ideals in their life, while others either took it for granted or did not consider it paramount.

But there's more! When asked what was more important, wealth or happiness, all said happiness. Of course. But when probed further, as to how much wealth they would forgo to achieve 'happiness', the answer never amounted to more than play money. Leftovers. So next time you hear a wealthy person saying money doesn't buy happiness, treat them with the same suspicion you reserve for the supermodel who says she envies fat people because they are jolly.

The point to all this is that our lives are made up of programmed responses. We invariably respond with answer B to question A. We invariably think X if someone suggests Y. Often there is no sense or logic to our responses, we have just been conditioned to respond that way.

The Centenarian Test is designed to short-circuit those conditioned answers. And because you are the only person who will ever know your answers, you can be as far-reaching as you dare. All you need is a blanket, a large pad and a felt pen or thick-leaded pencil.

The Centenarian Test

Go somewhere quiet where you will not be disturbed. If it's convenient, place a blanket over your lap – as some elderly people do.

- Tell yourself you have all the time in the world.

- After a couple of minutes of relaxing, listening to the sound of your breathing, and moving towards Deep Calm, close your eyes and let your imagination run wild.

- Imagine you were born over a century ago. Just before the 1900s arrived. Imagine what it would have been like to have been a child then. The things you would have seen, the things you would have heard, the clothes you would have worn. Would they be hot and uncomfortable? What would be the tastes and smells of that time? Cooking bread? Burning wax? You were a child then.

- Now, you're over 100 years old. And, like many centenarians, you're still independent and in full control of your faculties.

- With no 'future pressures' on your agenda, you think back over the life you've just led. Looking back. Reviewing. Thinking what made you happy, satisfied, fulfilled.

- What were the things you thought most important? Position? Wealth? Relationships? Was it that you spent your best time with your children, or fostering your relationships? Was it that you made a difference to the world at large, or in your immediate circles? What is most important to you now?

- Write these things down as they come to mind.

You should discover some interesting things about your core priorities and values by performing this test. It is simple, enjoyable and revealing. Moreover, you can conduct it many times – especially as you enter the different phases of your life. You will find it becomes more revealing each time.

Your conclusion as to what is most important in your life will probably not involve your job or your real estate portfolio. It may very well relate to making a difference in your world, or having developed and nurtured good relationships with those close to you. You might draw satisfaction from the fact that you developed many life-enriching skills, or wrote a cookbook, or circumnavigated the globe. But it may equally be that you had a rich and fulfilling life simply because your children grew up to be healthy and happy people.

Prepare to be surprised.

Each person is different. Each person has different values and different core needs. And even though these may vary from one life stage to the next, the deep underlying ones are usually with you forever. Whether you recognise them or not.

Now, having established what is important in your life, you are ready to use this information to shape your days ahead.

Your map of life One of the characteristics I've sometimes admired in others is an absolute commitment to an ideal. When this exists, life has purpose for them. They know their direction. Decisions are easier to make. They have a set of values that takes the guesswork out of morality and principles. And even if that ideal involves tough disciplines and denial, life seems easier. This is why some people find calm and contentment in asceticism. And in institutions. And fighting for causes.

Total commitment has other virtues as well. It makes for powerful leadership, especially if the individual concerned has the ability to communicate this sense of commitment to others. And when the commitment and ideals are shared, relationships are strengthened. Hence, you often find mismatched couples in satisfying relationships while they have shared ideals, such as raising children; then, when the children grow up, they grow apart.

Total commitment is foreign to most of us. Even when we become obsessed about a cause, or work slavishly towards certain goals, our drive usually falls way short of absolute commitment. Total commitment – or 'purpose', as some refer to it – comes from holistic ideals. Ideals that are so central to your being that you never have to think about them (once they have been identified). Using techniques such as the Centenarian Test helps you to identify your values and priorities, before you turn them into ideals.

When you have done this you have a road map for life.

If the Consequences you design for yourself fit neatly onto this road map, they are dramatically easier to accomplish.

The need for persistence

Nothing in the world can take the place of persistence. Talent will not; nothing in the world is more common than unsuccessful men with talent. Genius will not; unrewarded genius is a proverb. Education will not; the world is full of educated derelicts. Persistence and determination alone are omnipotent.

Calvin Coolidge

While I have been working on this book I have been conscious of the fact that most of what I have been writing about are activities of the mind – beliefs, attitudes, ways of using your own thought processes.

All of this may tend to suggest that extraordinary levels of achievement are very easy to realise. It is human nature to seek easy answers. In this age of instant gratification, this desire is even more pronounced. The idea that you can access all of life's opportunities and solve all of life's problems just by adopting certain mental postures is very seductive. But potentially misleading.

While we can accept that the mind is the deliverer of all human power and capability, we must not overlook the fundamental of achievement – that is, that every great achievement involves persistence. All things being equal, the greater the persistence, the greater the result.

Of all the successful people I have met over the years, none sought the easy answer. None. Without exception, they made immense physical, emotional, intellectual and spiritual investments in their capabilities.

The yogi who is so calm that he can slow his breathing rate and heartbeat to almost comatose levels does not attain this ability by using his mind alone. It requires long hours of regular physical and mental discipline.

The Chi Kung master who can overcome illness and endure almost unthinkable physical discomforts, does not do so by adopting mental attitudes alone. It takes years of difficult physical training and sacrifice.

When a great sportsperson or businessperson performs or achieves on an ongoing basis, it will usually be because of a combination of two factors: technique, and experience or practice.

The second of these, experience or practice (which can be one and the same), is not to be dismissed. When you have performed the same action over and over again, it becomes effortless. The moment the hurdler thinks about the hurdle in front, they lose the race. You perform best when you don't have to think about how you're performing. You do it unconsciously. This ability to perform an action unconsciously is vital. Some people do it through repetitive action, others do it through mental rehearsal; but it must be done. Then you can concentrate on approaching what you do from a calm state.

The fact that books like this tend to highlight the exceptions – the people who triumph over illnesses by using mental or unorthodox practices, or who achieve amazing things using a modicum of exertion – can sometimes create the illusion that no persistence is required. If you were to take that message from this book, I would be disappointed.

Because anything worth achieving is worth persevering with.

So far, you've discovered that:

- **Your greatest power and your maximum potential come from your calm centre.**

- **You have a choice of techniques that can take you to your calm centre and the experience of Deep Calm.**

- **From this Deep Calm state, you can achieve extraordinary things.**

- **By combining this with the Success Formula, you can achieve anything.**

- **Take this further and include the Calm Inspiration Cycle, and you will discover the most inspired solutions you are humanly capable of – at that particular moment – 100 percent of the time.**

8

APPLICATIONS
OF DEEP CALM

*There is a specific state of calm you
can use to aid healing, longevity,
prosperity and spiritual awareness.
It is called Deep Calm . . .*

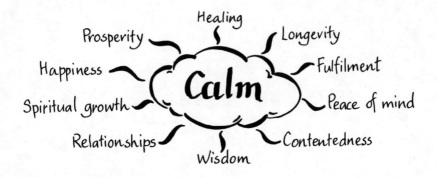

When you combine the state of Deep Calm with the Success Formula (page 183), you can achieve almost anything you set your mind to.

The vital element of this formula is an attribute we call 'i' – a beyond-the-ordinary level of inspiration or creativity, which is the product of the Calm Inspiration Cycle. The power of this process stems from the fact that you use *all* of your resources. Even if you are unaware of these, they do exist and they are powerful beyond your most ambitious expectations. They include all the innate wisdom and information you may not even have known you possessed, or had long since 'forgotten'. But, more importantly, when you are in tune with those resources, you intuitively understand what is the ideal solution for the *whole* you: your emotions, hidden desires, health, unique ways of thinking, values and belief systems.

No other human, or group of humans, has this insight into your strengths and your needs. No medical practitioner, psychologist, molecular biologist, priest, guru, spiritual leader, friend, relative or partner. When it comes to you, and what makes you tick, you will always know more. Infinitely more. Somewhere within you is this knowledge.

Being able to access it means you can also access certain abilities so astounding that some may see them as superhuman. They are not superhuman, of course; it's just that most people do not know how to access them. The only way you can access them with any degree of predictability is by going to your calm centre and relaxing into a state of Deep Calm. Even if you are not aware of it yet, you are getting close to the stage where you have the ability to do this. Now that you know the formula to finding inspired solutions to life's issues, you can apply it to any situation.

Calm for wellness and longevity

[You] can do more for your own health and wellbeing than any doctor, any hospital, any drug, any exotic medical advice.

US Surgeon General's report, 1979

There are some strange conceptions out there about who is responsible for the maintenance of our health. From a legal point of view this is fairly clear-cut – so I draw your attention to the disclaimer at the front of this book. The reason such a disclaimer is necessary is twofold. The first is health politics: the hard-won concession that only a medical 'authority' is qualified to offer advice in relation to your health (if they have insurance). The second stems from a fear that you will unquestioningly accept everything you read in a book such as this.

At the risk of appearing subversive, I want to make it clear that the master of my health and wellness is me. You might decide that the master of *your* health and wellness is . . . *you*. As far as I am concerned, that makes a lot of sense, but it is a decision for you to make. Whichever way you decide – retain the responsibility, or hand it over to someone else – you will have exercised your control and choice. And that is the point of this book.

There are also many strange conceptions about the nature of health. Some tend to think of becoming healthy as a goal, like a university doctorate – something you work towards, attain, then carry with you for the rest of your life. Some see it as a chore, something that has to be worked on, but which offers little satisfaction in its own right. Some see it as a remote and unfamiliar ideal. And others barely give it a second thought.

Health is a dynamic process. Sometimes it's good, sometimes not so good. For the state of good health to become a permanent part of your consciousness, it must be nourished and enjoyed on an ongoing basis. The key word here is 'enjoyed'. Good health can only be enjoyed when it is your creation. When you surrender the responsibility for your health and wellbeing to third parties – doctors, gurus, therapists – you give away much of the efficacy and all of the pleasure of it.

You probably don't need me to give you reasons why wellness is desirable. But here's one that is usually overlooked: it feels good! You feel alive. You appreciate life more. You live better, love better, see the humorous side of your world. All of your capabilities are increased. And, if you make a habit of wellness, you begin to see through the sophisticated veneer of your lifestyle. Suddenly, you begin to appreciate the simple pleasures – the pleasures of exercise, fresh air, fresh food, sound sleep, love, nature, simplicity and selflessness.

So, what are the steps to wellness?

To begin with, your health involves much more than your body. It involves every thought you have, as well as your relationships with those close to you and the world at large. If you nourish these, and get pleasure from them, you enhance not only your health, but your entire being. Wellness and longevity can be enhanced by concentrating on only six areas:

(i)   Look after your diet

(ii) Enjoy exercise

(iii) Develop a positive attitude

(iv) Love what you do

(v)   Help others

(vi) Learn to become calm.

You may already have thought of another three or four things that could be added to this list. But let me show you how they can all be reduced to these six simple steps.

(i) Look after your diet

Diet plays a major role in how you feel. It influences how you deal with the stresses and strains of life. To put it simply, too many stimulating foods, such as coffee, tea, sugar, alcohol, refined and pre-served foods, can leave you with an ongoing feeling of tension.

As well, diet is the single greatest influence on your state of health. It is estimated that more than 50 percent of the diagnosed illnesses in the United States have a direct relationship with dietary issues. These include alcoholism, diabetes, obesity, bulimia, anorexia, allergies, mal-nutrition and hypertension. In addition to this, we have an almost endless array of other conditions, for which diet is either the culprit or the prime suspect. These range from migraine, depression, chronic fatigue, cancer and heart disease all the way through to backache. It is easy, then, to accept the conclusion of the relatively conservative US Surgeon General, in his 1988 report, that nutrition is a factor in almost 70 percent of deaths in the community.

That's the negative side of nutrition.

On the positive side, some estimate that up to 90 percent of car-diovascular disease, cancers and other forms of degenerative illness could be prevented, or at least delayed, simply by adopting dietary measures – improved nutrition, better food combinations and mod-eration of the toxic elements in your diet.

This is easy to say, I know, but how easy is it to accomplish? Surprisingly easy, if you adopt two very simple sets of principles. The first relates to food balances.

When you were a child, you were taught the major food groups and advised to adjust your diet according to certain ratios within these groups. That served its purpose as a safeguard against malnutri-tion. But as a formula to help you become calm and enhance your wellness, in an over-refined, additive-enriched world, it leaves some-thing to be desired. That is why we need a simpler and more meaningful formula.

In the East, you will find the main food categories are sometimes reduced to two – Yin and Yang (in Chinese philosophy), Shiva and Shakti (in the Indian tradition). These almost correspond to the Western categorisation of acid-forming foods and alkaline-forming foods. Acid-forming foods leave an acidic residue after they have been exhausted in the stomach. Conversely, alkaline-forming foods leave an alkaline residue.

A common element in most states of ill-health is that the body's fluids (blood, lymph and saliva) are too acidic. It is widely understood that a concentration of acid in your system has an adverse effect on tissues and cells. Invariably, acidity has a dietary connection, and is usually caused by consuming too much animal protein, refined foods or junk food. The way you counter it, or prevent it, is by consuming more alkaline-forming foods. The accepted ratio you should strive to maintain in your diet is 80:20, 80 percent alkaline-forming foods to 20 percent acid-forming foods.

Food influences mood

It is interesting to observe that alkaline–acid ratios in your diet have a pronounced effect on your mood.

Alkaline-forming foods tend to encourage calm. Acid-forming foods tend to produce unrest.

The converse of this also applies: your state of calm influences your acid–alkaline balance. Slow, relaxed breathing encourages alkaline conditions, while tense, shallow breaths generate acid.

So, which is which?

All processed, fried, salty, preserved foods are acid forming. As are all animal products – meat, fish, poultry and dairy products (although butter and buttermilk are sometimes listed in the alkaline category). All uncooked fresh vegetables and fruits are alkaline forming.

The alkaline-forming properties of fruits and vegetables – particularly when raw – are considered an important part of many healing regimes. It's said, for example, that they assist the pancreas to produce certain enzymes that help in the fight against cancer.

The health benefits of consuming larger quantities of vegetables and fruit are unmistakeable. Studies consistently find that you more than double your risk of most types of cancer if your diet is low in fruit and vegetables. And these findings are remarkably similar when applied to other degenerative illnesses such as heart disease.

You can correct this dietary imbalance by applying the 80:20 formula. Maintain the ratio of 80:20 between alkaline- and acid-forming foods and you will not only feel better for it, you will be maintaining your wellness at the same time.

Alkaline-forming foods	Acid-forming foods
All fresh vegetables	All meat, fish, poultry
All fresh fruits	Eggs and most dairy products
Whole rice and whole flour	Wheat bran, refined flour, seeds
Millet	Sugar, salt, pepper
Molasses	Coffee, tea, carbonated drinks, alcohol
Dried fruits	Processed, refined and canned foods
Apple cider vinegar	Vinegar (distilled)
Most things that grow	Most things in packets

The second dietary principle that relates to calm and wellness involves a simple piece of philosophy. It relates to holism, as opposed to reductionism (see page 74 for more on this distinction). Nowhere is a holistic approach more important than when it comes to food.

The principle underlying it is very simple. Foods are like people. If you dissect a person, throw away all those yucky internal organs, then reconstitute the remaining parts, you would end up with something that may look passably like a real person – from a distance – but would hardly function like one. That sounds extreme, I know, but we treat our foods like this every day.

Take the example of bread. First we refine the flour and remove all its nutrients. Then, realising the severity of our actions, we try to compensate by throwing in a bit of manufactured folic acid and protein powder, a handful of wheat bran and a few assorted seeds. We then call this reconstruction 'wholewheat', and expect it to function like a real food. Which, of course, it doesn't. It's food in theory and intention, but not in nutrition. This is a reductionist view of foods. It does not take into account all the subtleties and fine balances – within the food and within the digestive system – that have evolved over eons.

So much of our daily diet consists of these quasi-scientific reconstructions. Homogenising milk breaks up the fat molecules – ostensibly for health reasons but often in fact for economic or handling reasons – and distributes them throughout the milk so that the body cannot process them in the normal way. Maybe you take your milk differently: reduced to a powder, stripped of all the dairy fats, then mixed with water and put in a cardboard pack. Skim milk. A man-made reconstruction. And an offence against the principles of wholefoods. But we 'need' it because we've been told to remove fats from our diets.

The only drawback is that some researchers have recently concluded that whole milk may actually be an aid to weight reduction! Whole milk contains conjugated linoleic acid (CLA) which, it is believed, reduces protein degradation and thus lessens body fat in both animals and humans. Many athletes now take CLA supplements to force glucose into their muscle cells and connective tissues instead of allowing it to turn into fat. The irony! Perhaps you should take more notice of your local *barista* when he says, '*Il latte scremato in un cappucino é abominevole!!*' ('Skim milk in a cappuccino is an abomination!')

Taking a wholefood approach to your diet is easy. Wherever possible, choose foods that are as close as possible to the way nature intended them to be – not canned, refined, overcooked or overspiced. Then you'll discover how food can help you become calm . . . and healthy.

Finally, diet is more than food. There is also the diet of the mind.

This involves your consumption of information and entertainment. Choose well, and your entire wellbeing is enhanced.

(ii) Enjoy exercise

Whether you give in to it or not, you do have a natural inclination to exercise from time to time. Apart from satisfying a natural inclination, this has a number of benefits in how you feel.

When a stressful situation arises, activity in the sympathetic nervous system is increased: your muscles tense, your heart rate increases, anxiety hormones are secreted, blood sugar levels rise, and so on. Your alert state prevails until you expend some serious energy – such as through exercise. Physical activity increases the levels of endorphins in your system which tend to make you calmer, more relaxed and more pleasant – and help to counteract anger and depression. As well, exercise serves the very useful purpose of suspending thought and vocalisation by substituting a simple, physical activity.

This is why regular exercise calms the nerves, induces a restful feeling, helps you to sleep better, and enhances your long-term ability to deal with stressful situations. So physical exercise is not only beneficial to your cardiovascular fitness, it also improves your mood and overall mental health.

However, while some think of exercise as a chore, it's important to learn to enjoy it for its own sake. The way to do this is to stop thinking of it as a therapy, and start thinking of it as an indulgence. This is your own private time. Escape time. Unwinding time. Relaxing time. Luxuriating in your own company time. The fact that you have 20–45 minutes to spend, with no other objective but taking care of your body and state of mind is, by any measure, a luxury. Yes, even an indulgence. When you can view it this way, your whole perspective on exercise begins to change.

No doubt you've heard of the 'runner's high', the euphoric feeling that can arise from extended periods of exercise. Long-distance runners can become quite addicted to this feeling, which results from the release of endorphins and natural steroids into the bloodstream, usually at about the same rate that lactic acid concentration builds (the pain-reducing properties of the former balancing the pain-producing properties of the latter). If you're depending on this runner's high to help you enjoy exercise, be prepared for some hard work – it doesn't cut in until you approach the pain barrier, typically after an hour or so of intense exercise.

If you do not have an exercise program at the moment, you're in good company. In some countries, around 80 percent of the population do not. But you are missing out on a lot by not having one.

Choosing the right program is not something to lose sleep over. While any form of exercise will suffice, an easy choice is walking. There are other choices, of course. If you are not suffering any serious medical conditions (have a check-up if you're unsure), a calm exercise program might consist of about five workouts a week, each lasting for 20–45 minutes, depending on the type of exercise.

Let's look at a few nice relaxing possibilities:

- Walk for 45 minutes, or until you get to where you want to go.

- Run for 25 minutes, or longer if you're attracted to that 'runner's high'.

- Swim for 25 minutes, or until you run out of laps.

- Cycle (at a reasonable speed) for 45 minutes.

- Perform aerobics for 25 minutes, or until the tape runs out.

- Dance for as long as your heart desires.

Generally, the ideal exercise is considered to be a minimum of 20 minutes – at a level where you feel warm and breathe more heavily than usual – at least three, preferably five, times a week.

If you have no particular inclination towards any type of exercise, let me return to my original suggestion: walk. It's easy, portable, and possibly the most relaxing exercise program available. Do it in a place that gives you pleasure, and the benefits multiply. My recommendation is five times a week, for 30–45 minutes. Treat it as an indulgence, enjoy it, and it will help you attain a longer, healthier, happier and more productive life.

I do urge you to adopt an exercise program. There is a risk involved when you believe that the mind is the greatest healer, and that a clear direction and a positive attitude is all it takes to make your way through life. The risk is that, by placing our faith in such intangibles, we overlook the single most important tangible in our lives – the physical reality of our own bodies.

Being aware of your body, and knowing how to keep it functioning effectively, is an essential element of your mental and spiritual development.

(iii) Develop a positive attitude

Most optimists succeed, all pessimists fail

One of the earliest discoveries we make in life is that it is easier to complain about problems than it is to offer solutions. As a result we see large parts of our society obsessed with what is wrong. This applies not only to protest movements, but also to members of the clergy, teaching, politics and most particularly the media.

It requires very little insight, effort or character to be able to highlight the wrongs of life. The real challenge is to present constructive possibilities.

Once you make a habit of seeing life from a positive perspective, this becomes easy.

If you've ever seen the film *Pollyanna*, you will recall a game the characters played in times of adversity. They called it the Glad Game. The object of the Glad Game was to try to find something about every situation to be glad about: easy during good times, but requiring more creativity during difficult times.

Some cynics say that positive thinking is a con; that all the positive attitude in the world won't help you overcome illness or succeed in areas where you would otherwise fail.

Let me show you why they're wrong.

For a start, optimism is its own reward. It helps overcome depression and ill-feeling, and generally makes you feel good about life. Optimism has a direct link with health and longevity. For people under 60 years of age, there is a clear correlation between positive attitude and good health.

It has often been said that attitude is less important after 60 years of age. However, there has been at least one major study of people aged between 55 and 65 years, tracking their progress over a 20-year period. It was shown, once again, that attitude plays a vital role – with those who were considered most optimistic being many times more likely to remain alive and well than those considered the most pessimistic. Those who rated highest on the 'optimism' scale were more likely to assume responsibility for their health, and to maintain better diet and exercise programs. Which came first? Who cares?

It is now fairly widely established that having a positive mental attitude not only enhances your immune system and circulation, but also significantly reduces your risk of encountering an accident or 'bad luck'.

If you ask the more progressive immunologists for the best prescription against cancer, most will volunteer diet and/or optimism. As a predictor of longevity, a positive or optimistic attitude is so important that many believe it has more bearing than any of the risk factors conventionally cited, including smoking, a sedentary lifestyle, diet and genetics.

However, it is important that optimism is seen not just as an expectation of certain outcomes, but as a real commitment to positive behaviour and attitudes. In other words, optimism is active, not passive.

> *Beware the man that laughs and his belly does not jiggle.*
> Confucius

Closely aligned with optimism and a positive attitude is laughter. Or the ability to bring happiness to your life by seeing the fun and amusing side of it.

When your body is under stress, your adrenal glands produce a steroid called cortisol, which is designed to calm you down. Among other things, it is known that too much cortisol can decrease the effectiveness of your immune system, thus making you vulnerable to illness and disease. Just by laughing, you reduce the production of cortisol and cause your endocrine system to release a range of neurochemicals which relax the body, suppress pain, aid digestion and improve blood flow.

So, it pays to look for the humorous side of life. Sometimes this is difficult but, as with the Glad Game, you can make an entertainment of finding the lighter side of life.

Finally, a tense frame of mind invariably encourages a negative perspective on life. The more you succumb to the tensions of the day, the bleaker life appears. When you maintain a state of inner calm, you automatically develop a positive attitude towards life. Maintain the calm, and you maintain the positive attitude.

(iv) Love what you do

Technically, this should probably be included under the heading of 'Develop a positive attitude'. However, this point is so important to your enjoyment of life and your sense of fulfilment, that it really deserves its own category.

How would you like to work as a talk show host? Being driven around in stretch limousines, every whim taken care of, on everybody's A list, the media hanging off your every word. Wouldn't you just love all that?

How about something a little less stratospheric? How would you like to be living on a tropical island paradise? Tahiti, Hawaii, the Seychelles – pick a paradise. Slinking about in a sarong all day, not a care in the world, and no decisions to make other than which beach you're going to lie on this morning, what tropical fruit you're going to eat at lunch. Wouldn't you love to live like that?

Obviously, very few of us get to experience lifestyles such as these, and if we did, we probably wouldn't think of them as being so idyllic. Nevertheless, even if you can't manage to live the life you'd love to live, or to work in the job you'd love to have, you can always learn to love the life you're already living.

Imagine discovering a simple art to learning to love what you do – whatever it is you do. There is. Whether this is the work you do, the parents you live with, or the luck you've been dealt, it can be a thoroughly satisfying and fulfilling activity.

Just by using a simple technique.

One of the beauties of Zen philosophy is the way it encourages you to concentrate on making the most of NOW, by occupying yourself completely in the moment. This applies not only to meditation and martial arts, but to all of life's activities – working, dining, walking, reading, everything. Being able to concentrate this way can turn an ordinary, everyday activity into a meditation (almost). It can increase efficiency and make time fly. It can be calming.

Here is a simple technique you can use to help you learn to love what you do – whatever it is that you do.

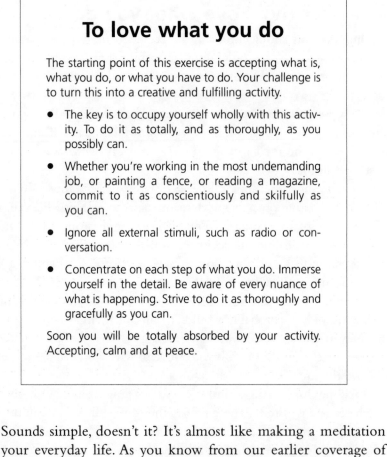

To love what you do

The starting point of this exercise is accepting what is, what you do, or what you have to do. Your challenge is to turn this into a creative and fulfilling activity.

- The key is to occupy yourself wholly with this activity. To do it as totally, and as thoroughly, as you possibly can.

- Whether you're working in the most undemanding job, or painting a fence, or reading a magazine, commit to it as conscientiously and skilfully as you can.

- Ignore all external stimuli, such as radio or conversation.

- Concentrate on each step of what you do. Immerse yourself in the detail. Be aware of every nuance of what is happening. Strive to do it as thoroughly and gracefully as you can.

Soon you will be totally absorbed by your activity. Accepting, calm and at peace.

Sounds simple, doesn't it? It's almost like making a meditation of your everyday life. As you know from our earlier coverage of meditation, dividing your attention creates tension, while concentrating your attention on only one thing is both calming and fulfilling. And it places you in complete control of what you do.

Another way of learning to love what you do is being able to view it in terms of making a difference. I have mentioned this before: having purpose in your life; being able, through what you do, to make a difference – to yourself, your family, the world around you – is the most satisfying and enriching way to approach any activity in life.

As you read through the next section, you will see how loving what you do and helping others are closely related.

(v) Help others

Spread love everywhere you go . . . first of all in your own house. Give love to your children, to your wife or husband, to a next-door neighbour . . . let no-one ever come to you without leaving better and happier. Be the living expression of God's kindness; kindness in your face, kindness in your eyes, kindness in your smile, kindness in your warm greeting.

Mother Teresa

It's a jungle out there. And in this help-yourself world, you have to be ultra-focused on your own needs in order to achieve anything of substance. This is why it's easy to lose sight of the fact that we're all playing individual roles in a much larger story. While each of us may be as unique as any fingerprint or snowflake, we are also like one pixel on a vast screen. If, as many physicists now believe, there is truth in the radical theory that there are as many universes as there are people, that means there are billions of people presently playing a role in *your* particular universe. Think of the responsibility.

I want to share my belief about the responsibility of success, good fortune and prosperity (all types of prosperity, not just financial) – a belief shared by all the successful people I've ever met and admired. The more successful and accomplished you become, and the more confidence, wisdom and understanding you accumulate, the more you are obliged to hand back.

Who are you obliged to? Just to yourself; not another soul. Moreover, it is not even a moral obligation (at least, not as far as I know), it is simply one of equity; of fairness and balance. You can read 'karma' into that statement if you wish. I don't think that is my intention, though. One can never be sure about these things, but I think I mean it in a more self-serving way. I think I mean that you owe it to your own continued development to hand back some of your confidence, wisdom and understanding. Or, as it was once explained to me: you cannot be the master unless you accept the students.

What I am suggesting is that you do this for selfish reasons. For your own satisfaction. Take time out for generosity. Share your good fortune. Find the good in others. Remember great people help others to become great, while small people try to hold others back. There is no more effective way to rise above your own limitations. Besides, one of the most satisfying ways of relieving your own stress and depression is to make a habit of helping others to relieve theirs.

When you immerse yourself in helping another individual, you overcome the self-centred nature of your own stresses and anxieties; you reduce the feeling of isolation that often accompanies them. After helping others, you should experience a sense of elation and accomplishment; in the longer term, this leads to feelings of peace and power. Seek out opportunities to help others. For your own sake.

Finally, helping others engenders the most irreplaceable of all emotions – love.

> *You will find as you look back upon your life that the moments when you have truly lived are the moments when you have done things in the spirit of love.*
>
> Henry Drummond

Love means infinitely more than you'd assume from the classic sentimental definition. It is a positive, healing, calming form of energy. To be effective, though, it must be directed inwards as much as outwards.

It starts from deep inside, with a love and acceptance of yourself, what you are and what you have done. This may not be an easy first step. For some, it will involve forgiveness for what is or what has passed – for being unsuccessful, uncaring, dishonest, lonely, ill or unattractive. For others, it will involve forgiveness for the things you blame yourself for, are angry about, or regret. Forgiveness of this nature requires more than just words and sentiments, it requires your total sincerity.

To love what you are

If you think of love as a form of energy, which in quiet moments you can direct inwards to heal or to give pleasure, you'll begin to discover it's something you can really feel.

- Sit quietly, practising any of the Step 2 or Step 3 techniques given on pages 130–70 until you are deeply relaxed. Tell yourself you have all the time in the world.

- Feel yourself surrounded by a halo of warm energy. Imagine it's a positive energy. A peaceful, loving energy that asks nothing of you, except that you accept it.

- It makes you smile!

- Feel the smile on your face as you draw that energy inwards. Feel the smile helping your facial muscles to relax. Feel the smile warming and embracing your body. Permeating your body with a healing, forgiving, undemanding energy. This is love at its most pure.

- Luxuriate in it . . .

Add this brief exercise to your regular meditation or relaxation program, and take pleasure in the change it brings.

Once you can love and accept your own self, you can start to direct it outwards. Think of it as a positive energy. Radiate it indiscriminately. To those close to you, to the people you work with, to the people you come in contact with on a daily basis.

Forget all those sentimental precepts about loving, and *radiate*. Then – and this is equally important – accept it when it is reciprocated.

(vi) Learn to become calm

As a form of preventative therapy, Deep Calm (or meditation) rates alongside diet and exercise. It can have the most profound effect on your mood and state of mind – particularly if you've adopted it as part of your lifestyle. It is no secret that altering your state of consciousness through meditation can do more than affect your immediate health: it has been shown to extend human life and to limit, or even reverse, age-related degeneration.

To show definitively that meditation extends life expectancy is not a simple task, though. For a start, such studies have to span many years, and so many other factors need to be ruled out. Nevertheless, I know of at least one study that was conducted in a nursing home for the elderly. One group was taught how to meditate, the other was taught conventional relaxation techniques. Among the meditating group, the improvement – in general health, mobility, mood and mental agility – was pronounced; significantly better than the other group. And the survival rate of the meditating group over the 6-year period of the study was 100 percent, whereas the other group was notably less fortunate.

Studies such as this show a clear link between meditation, health and longevity. We know, for example, that regular meditation helps to lower your blood pressure and cholesterol levels. We know it retards the ageing process (by boosting the immune system and reducing the production of free radicals). We also know that people who meditate regularly have lower rates of heart disease, tumours and nervous illnesses. Is this proof of increased life expectancy? If you're a scientist, maybe not. If you're like most people I know, it's proof enough. More than enough.

When you try Deep Calm for yourself, there will be no question.

One more thing. The meditative state produces a range of mood-enhancing neurochemicals that not only help you to feel on top of the world (bliss is a word that is often used), but also help to reverse the negative effects of stress.

What about longevity?

This morning on the radio, I heard a scientist suggesting that ours could be the last mortal generation. He said that death could become a thing of the past for people born today, and that immortality would soon be a scientific possibility.

Not long after that I read an interview with Quentin Crisp. At 90, he was bemoaning the fact that his body had worn out, and that for him death could not come quickly enough.

I choose not to speculate on the theoretical lifespan of a human being. Immortality is probably a bit ambitious for most people. So, too, is living for 130-odd years. But there would be few among us who would not be grateful for another decade or so. Medical researchers tell us we can extend our lives by up to 14 years (on average), simply by making a few lifestyle changes. Surely this is incentive enough to make you want to take a serious look at your lifestyle.

Let's look at what we know about longevity.

The average life expectancy of a person in most countries is increasing. You might think that this is the result of medical intervention helping older people to live longer. However, this is not necessarily so. In recent years, increases in life expectancy have been brought about largely by improved diet and reduced infant mortality (deaths from childhood diseases decreased by 90 percent between 1850 and 1950).

You've probably heard commentators saying that the surest recipe for living to a ripe old age is to choose the right parents. However, at best, genetics adds only another 3 years to the life expectancy. This is not to say that people who do live to a ripe old age do not have strong genetics working in their favour; they do.

But, apart from choosing your parents wisely and being born a woman (to benefit from the longer life expectancy of women), what can you do to extend your life in a fulfilling and meaningful way?

A recent study of centenarians revealed only one attribute that all of them shared: an ability to dispense with stressful situations with an optimist outlook ('I've got plans').

What else do we know?

- The life expectancy of vegetarians tends to be some years longer than non-vegetarians (although precise figures vary from country to country).

- The life expectancy of people who eat three to five servings of fruit and vegetables a day is substantially longer than that of those who don't.

- Members of certain religious communities who pray and abstain from alcohol and coffee live years longer than members of the wider community – on average.

- The life expectancy of people who meditate, people who exercise, and people who have positive attitudes are all many years longer than for those who don't – on average.

Of course none of this would mean a thing if all these long-lived people were having a miserable time of it. But their experience is the opposite of that.

Take meditation. At all stages of their life, most meditators rate their quality of life as higher than do their non-meditating counterparts. This rating involves a range of subjective factors, including contentedness, vitality and feelings of hope.

I would also be prepared to wager that the subjective experience of those who exercise, those who have a positive attitude and those who are vegetarian would likewise result in a higher assessment of their quality of life.

Clearly, enhanced quality of life combined with an extended lifespan is an objective worth striving for. Learning to love being calm, good food, refreshing exercise and the world around you is a small price to pay.

Healing yourself

If you break your leg or cut your arm, there are accepted procedures you would expect to follow to assist with its healing. These are well-defined interventions that involve splints, plaster casts, pain control, stitches and the like.

However, when the ailment is more organic – particularly when it involves painful, life-threatening or degenerative conditions – the solutions are not so clear-cut. Healing in these types of conditions often involves more than physical intervention.

Healing is among the most personal of all activities in life. And, even if you're surrounded by the most caring and understanding support group, even if you have the best medical services in the world, it is largely a solo effort. What happens inside your head has a profound influence on what happens to the rest of your body.

Modern medicine has been slow to acknowledge this. The very notion that a patient's thoughts and feelings could dictate the outcome of their treatment is anathema to the practice of most doctors and scientists. How can they control it? You will have heard the scorn heaped on certain treatments and therapies: 'This is nonsense; it's the placebo effect'. (A placebo is a fake treatment, such as a sugar pill, provided instead of the real one in clinical experiments designed to test the efficacy of a drug or therapy. Although it is widely accepted by the medical community, the very concept seems cynical and contrary to the nature of healing. Surely if a medical researcher gets to the stage where he believes drug X will work, then simply *pretends* to issue this to half an experiment's subjects, he is denying those people his best attempts to heal. What would Hippocrates say about that?)

However, the reason placebos exist is that medical researchers know that patient expectation will influence the outcome of their experiments. They know this. So, when someone says, 'It's only the placebo effect,' what they usually mean is that the therapy didn't work because of the intrinsic value of the therapy, it only worked because the patient *thought* it was going to work. In other words, you're not really feeling well, you only *think* you're feeling well. Poor you.

This understanding of the power of thought is a cornerstone of medical research, yet it is not considered a credible part of healing. Why? Pure science is not remotely interested in what you think works best for you, or indeed what does work best for you; that is considered subjective and irrelevant. It is concerned only with the quantitative aspects of what will work for people regardless of their beliefs.

The fact is that the placebo effect works very effectively for large numbers of people involved in clinical experiments – often matching the effects of a drug, *including its side effects*. To my mind, this suggests that the placebo effect is worth nurturing. Think what it could save in drug costs each year! Think what could be achieved if the placebo was associated with miracle cures that hadn't yet been discovered!

'Half of you are going to take this new miracle drug that cures cancer, baldness and cellulite. The other half will receive a sugar pill (placebo). We're going to test the results in 6 months.'

Guess what would happen if *everyone* received the placebo! A large proportion of our group would start growing back their hair (or believing their hair was growing), cancers would shrink, and cellulite would smooth over. That's how the placebo effect works.

More importantly, that's how the mind works. Unfortunately, it's not scientifically acceptable because it depends on the recipient, not the input of the scientist or medical authority.

Thankfully, the mind of the individual is at last being recognised for the important role it can play in the health of that individual.

The healing power of the mind Not so long ago I had lunch with a very excited neurophysiologist. He and his researchers had made a remarkable discovery – that the human mind could be shown to actually bring about healing in the body. Noting the fact that I had not fallen off my chair over this disclosure, he wondered how I could remain so calm.

'Surely most people already know that,' I said.

'How could they? We've only just completed the experiment.'

But think about it: haven't you and I known about the potency of the mind all along? Haven't we always known that what you think, becomes; that if you think yourself well, you become well. Unfortunately, science moves much more slowly than ordinary humans in this respect.

The principle of mind–body healing is that attitude can play as important a role in the healing process as the organs. Once this is accepted, you must assume responsibility for your own health. You do this by ensuring that your focus extends beyond your illness or condition, and works on your attitudes, thought processes and lifestyle. Central to it are the centring skills we discover in, or that stem from, Deep Calm.

You might well wonder why modern medicine has taken so long to arrive at this principle – if indeed it has arrived. After all, your emotions are not remote, mystical experiences, but are distinctly physiological in nature. Not only do they influence your subjective experience, but every cell in your body as well. Every thought or emotion you have produces something known as a neuropeptide – a messenger molecule that travels from your brain in search of other specific cells (such as those that relate to your immune system) to team up with. Once this connection has taken place, there is a physical relationship between your brain cells and cells that perform other functions in your body.

It is fairly elementary biochemistry, therefore, that shows a clear physical link between your thought processes and your immune system.

When you're happy and relaxed, your body produces a range of healing chemicals – including serotonin (aids sleep, enhances mood and regulates aggression), melatonin (regulates sleep and improves immune response), interferon (fights infections, cancer, allergies and poisoning), and dopamine (brings pleasure). People who are happy and relaxed, *and meditate as well*, produce much higher levels of some of these chemicals.

On the other hand, when you're stressed and depressed, your body produces chemicals such as cortisol, histamines, adrenalin and nor-adrenalin, all of which are known to suppress the immune system. Stress is also known to reduce the number of helper T cells, which are one of the body's most important mechanisms for fighting disease.

By any measure, there is a clear physiological link between your thoughts and feelings and your state of health.

Yet, rather than try to exploit the possibilities inherent in this relationship, the focus of much medical research continues in the same vein. I have recently seen the results of a large scientific study into faith healing, which show only a weak connection between religion and spirituality and one's health. Anyone could have told them that. But instead of investing all that research effort in trying to discredit some fairly basic beliefs (which, I understand, was the motivation), wouldn't it have been more productive to explore how such beliefs could be used, or *modified*, to enhance health? After all, we know that faith and hope do help many people to overcome illness; how could we use these qualities to help more?

This mind–body connection in healing warrants more exploration than the fledgling psychoneuro-immunology (PNI) programs in operation today. It suggests that there should be a move away from the traditional doctor–patient hierarchy, towards more holistically orientated relationships that may or may not involve 'alternative' therapies. Strictly speaking, PNI is not much more than a psychological overlay on conventional medical therapies. A true holistic approach to healing would take into account the spiritual dimensions of the recipient as well.

So, if we accept that emotions produce quantifiable physiological effects, the question must be asked, which emotions produce which effects?

If you search for any scientific research on this, you'll find volumes of it focusing on the negative emotions and their effects on the immune system. Pessimism, anger and fear, for example, have been shown to be detrimental to health, particularly in the longer term.

But there are fewer significant studies addressing the converse of this: whether *positive* emotions – love, happiness, optimism – produce a positive effect on health. I can only surmise that the reason is a lack of incentive: as positive emotions do not constitute reproducible 'treatments', they are of lesser interest to the medical establishment, and are of even less interest to medical science's main benefactors, the pharmaceutical companies.

Fortunately, there are a few mavericks who have gone to the trouble of showing the connection. In one English study, it was shown that pleasant smells, such as the aroma of chocolate, or having pleasant thoughts, had a pronounced positive impact on the immune system – the body's immunoglobulins (proteins that fight infection) doubled within 20 minutes and remained at this level for at least 3 hours.

Unpleasant thoughts had the opposite effect.

The bottom line is that if your immune system is suppressed in any way, such as through ill health, depression or the stresses of every-day life, then positive emotions will help restore it.

The extremes of emotion

If we know that mood, emotion and thought have a direct and meas-urable influence on the body's immune system, does it follow that the more intense the mood, the greater will be the influence?

I read about a study conducted in this area in the early 1990s. The subjects of this experiment were well-trained Method actors, who specialised in producing intense moods and emotions for their roles.

When they acted out specific moods and emotions – genuinely experiencing these to some degree – they were tested for a range of immune system factors. The results confirmed that positive moods and emotions produced clear positive effects on their immune systems, while negative moods and emotions produced negative effects, suppressing their immune response.

Become a picture of health

- Go somewhere quiet, listen to your breathing, and allow yourself to ease into the state of Deep Calm. Tell yourself you have all the time in the world.

- In your imagination, picture yourself as calm, healthy and full of vitality.

- Pay attention to how well you look. Clear eyes, clean complexion, upright stance, the hint of a smile on your face.

- Pay attention to how well you sound. Your voice is clear, your breathing regular and deep. Perhaps other people comment on how well you look and sound.

- Next, pay attention to how well you *feel*. You feel alive, vibrant, eager to get on with the day. You feel like you have unlimited energy. You feel a loving, warm glow envelop you.

- Now, start pretending you are exactly like the person you are imagining. Act as if you really look, sound and feel exactly like that.

- Use the words you would use if you really were feeling the way you're pretending to feel. Even when you're not speaking, form words such as these in your mind.

- Finally, pretend that others see you as the calm, healthy, vital person you're pretending to be.

No great surprises there. But one of the real surprises came from the detail of this study. The effects on the immune system were not influenced by the (subjective) depth of the mood or emotion that the actor was experiencing. The immune system factors were affected – either positively or negatively – by even the most superficial portrayal of a mood or emotion. This led us to speculate that, since the intensity of emotion is not important to producing a positive immune response, and even a superficial enactment of a mood or emotion could produce this effect, maybe just *pretending* to be positive (or happy, or in love, or whatever) could produce the same effect.

It did.

And, while this study would be unlikely to stand up to the rigours of a fully-fledged clinical experiment, the indications are clear enough: simply by pretending to be happy, or contented, or well, you can bring about an ongoing positive effect on your immune system.

But you already knew that, didn't you?

The exercise outlined in the box on page 269 makes use of this knowledge.

A note of caution here: if you happen to be suffering from any medical condition, you may find this a powerful enhancement to your therapy. (And, even if it isn't, it will help you to feel better.) But it is possible that such a process could mask the symptoms which your therapist or practitioner will be looking for. I am obliged to point this out for, if your therapist or practitioner is to give an accurate diagnosis, you must be frank with them about your symptoms.

The positive effects of meditation

One of the simplest and surest ways of producing positive emotions and a positive frame of mind – and so keeping your immune system operating at its peak – is through meditation. When you meditate you actually reverse the stress process; your physiology virtually becomes the opposite of what it is when you're under pressure. For this reason meditation has become a popular addition to many healing programs, whether for physical trauma, disease or mental exhaustion.

There have been many studies conducted on the health benefits of meditation. Of particular interest is its effect on the immune system.

One of the hormones released by the body in stressful situations is cortisol. Its purpose is to restore your sense of calm after periods of stress, but in today's relentless world we seldom allow ourselves the necessary time for rest and restoration, so cortisol continues to be pumped into the bloodstream. This creates problems. Foremost among these is that it inhibits the immune system, making you vulnerable to illness or disease. Regular meditation puts a halt to this, either slowing or reversing this process; it is not uncommon to find cortisol levels dropping by 25 percent in experienced meditators. Even short-term meditators (with less than 3 years' experience) demonstrated significant improvements in their immune response.

There was a time when meditation and Western medicine were at opposite ends of the healing spectrum, as wide apart as shamanism and science. These days there is sufficient evidence — both clinical and anecdotal — to show that meditation is a powerful adjunct to most therapies. Many have discovered that extended periods of Deep Calm, when used in conjunction with other therapies, can greatly assist the healing process. As a result, you can now find meditation teachers affiliated with medical centres. By helping sufferers work their way through serious illnesses, these meditation teachers have brought hope to thousands who would otherwise have been regarded as hopeless cases. And by adding meditation programs to their treatments, the physicians have greatly enhanced the effectiveness of their treatments, at least on a subjective level.

Why does Deep Calm work this way?

As we've shown before, positive attitudes and emotions (by-products of meditation) enhance healing and reinforce the immune system. We also know that rest is a necessary part of the healing process, and meditation is probably the most profoundly restful state attainable.

The most compelling answer, however, may be even simpler than that. Regular practice of Deep Calm helps you to discard extraneous mental activity (thoughts) and to focus your mind on just one thing; the longer you meditate, the more proficient you become at focusing. If getting well is the major issue in your life, it helps to be able to channel all your effort into it. When you have the ability to focus, you can bring all your psychic energies to bear on this one task: restoring your health.

In addition, the psychological benefits of Deep Calm as an aid to healing are even more profound. It is a sure way to find peace, harmony and improved spirits at a time when all these are sorely needed.

Using calm to heal

Meditation or meditation-type practices are playing increasingly larger roles in more conventional healing practices. A great many mainstream therapists now encourage, or at least approve of, calming practices, recognising that Deep Calm, or meditation, is both physically and emotionally restorative.

When powerful healing is required, patients are encouraged by some therapists to spend many hours a day in meditation. What does this achieve?

The success stories are myriad. You have no doubt heard some of them yourself – as long as there are people with faith in the therapies, whatever they are, there will be success stories. You will find, though, that the practice of meditation is connected with most of them. But is it the meditation that heals, or the therapies it is aligned with?

I know of 'hopeless' cases where no other therapy was involved – so meditation had to be the means by which the person effected their own healing. I also know that if it were me in the firing line, I would be accepting whatever help I could get . . . Ultimately, though, you'll have to be the judge of what works best.

Of course, meditation is not the only complementary therapy being used in the treatment of life-threatening illnesses. Other therapies range from acupuncture to vitamin therapy and massage. They all have a role to play, and many are very successful in what they do.

One particular therapy closely aligned with meditation is Chi Kung, one of the four healing traditions of Chinese medicine. Its advocates claim that it heals by balancing and enhancing our natural healing resources. The successes attributed to Chi Kung are as extravagant as those attributed to meditation. However, buried in the hyperbole is a powerful healing force.

Chi, or Qi, means energy or life force. It is a concept that is widely accepted throughout Asia, the Middle East, and by most indigenous cultures. Chi Kung uses the focused mind to direct this internal

energy throughout the body. Directed towards troubled organs or tissue, this life force can be used as a healing technique for yourself or
for others. I have seen it used to heal tissue damage, and have a degree
of faith in its internal healing powers as well. Directed against an
opponent's body, it also becomes a powerful martial arts tool. I have
seen Chi Kung masters visibly move this Chi throughout their body
– like a ripple of energy moving beneath the flesh.

What follows is a showy piece of trivia, but it will serve as a simple
demonstration of a power that every human possesses, but few of us
realise we have, and even fewer believe we can apply. It is a demonstration of how easy it is to move energy through your body.

- Clench your left hand – rapidly and
  tightly – so that you feel the tension
  in your wrist and forearm muscles.

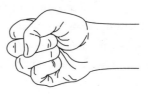

- Keep doing this until you can feel
  the strain in your arm and hand.

- After about 3 minutes of this, stop.

- Unfold your hand and lay it on your
  lap. Feel the tingling and energy?

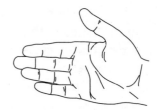

- Now, using nothing more than the
  power of your mind, transfer that
  tingling sensation to your right hand.

- Using only your thoughts – transfer it!

You will find that the transfer of energy (or, in this case, feeling)
from one part of your body to another – using nothing more than
the power of your thoughts – is incredibly simple. Anyone can do it.
Imagine doing this on a large scale. Imagine doing this to deliver
healing energy to a specific part of the body.

This is often how meditative techniques such as guided imagery are
used: the attention of the patient is taken to the body's trouble spot,
whereupon the patient is guided through an imagined healing or exci-
sion of the problem. While I know this practice is very powerful, and
is used by a great many therapists, I will not be encouraging it in this
book. This is for one reason only. I believe that guided imagery, when

it relates to a specific illness or condition, requires a trained guide. It is very possible for you to do this yourself. However, if your focus is not strong enough, you run the risk of dwelling on the negative, which could be counter-productive. Besides, your body unconsciously knows what it needs to heal itself better than you consciously do.

My preference is for meditation alone, without specific purpose, but beginning with a clear vision of yourself as healed, well and vibrant. In other words, a positive image of what you're working towards. Many great healing successes have come from this practice.

What will your physician say about this?

It would be naïve to suggest there is not some mainstream resistance, if not outright cynicism, towards therapies such as meditation and Chi Kung. I spent many years on the board of a surgical hospital, which was very much a part of the medical establishment, so I am acquainted with this resistance. I know that the few times I did speak about such healing practices, it was not taken all that seriously. But while we must respect the power of conventional medicine, we must also recognise its limitations. Sometimes these limitations can be destructive.

When you're sitting in a highly respected oncologist's office and they say there's nothing more they can do for you – you've got 12 months to live – you're in deep trouble. They have done much more than admit that conventional medicine has nothing more to offer: they have issued you with a highly damaging suggestion. If you accept their authority, you accept their prognosis; after all, they earn their reputation by being accurate with their predictions . . . don't they? You can see the paradox: their reputation rides on their ability to accurately predict their patient's demise, so they have a professional interest (theoretically speaking) in your keeping to schedule; you, in turn, are influenced by their reputation. Hence, you are negatively programmed.

In addition, such 'death deadlines' are notoriously anxiety-producing. And, while anxiety is of minor interest to the medical profession – which may have dismissed its importance since it has no organic function, and/or have written you off anyway – it is a destructive force in healing and should be dispensed with.

I mean no disrespect to oncologists when I point out these

problems. I would probably consult one if I were to find myself in this position. However we should recognise the programming power of prognoses such as these 'death deadlines' and seize the responsibility for our own health. Because you can be much more influential than other parties when it comes to matters of your own healing and longevity.

The role of the healer

If you have an acute condition, the sensible thing to do is to consult a physician. The last thing you want to be doing if you're bleeding, having a heart attack or you've got a chicken bone lodged in your throat is discussing the nature of healing and the subtle ramifications of holism.

As far as I am concerned, in acute situations there is no viable alternative to decisive action from a dedicated professional trained to respond to emergencies. Yet, with all the experience, intelligence, research and good intentions in the medical profession, it is disappointing to think that the direction of modern medicine often runs counter to the real spirit of healing.

When medical practitioners are besotted with their versions of what is real, and with scientific accuracy – neither of which has much relevance to your health – they end up focusing on the problem rather than the solution. This may not necessarily be in your best interest. You know from experience that if you're told you're sick, and what your symptoms are meant to be, you'll begin experiencing these symptoms. Sometimes your health will decline as a result. Yet, if you're continually reassured that there is hope, that these symptoms have meaning, and that 'if you do X, you will start feeling better' (as opposed to 'cured'), then those suggestions stand a very good chance of becoming self-fulfilling.

Some time ago, while I was clearing leaves in the garden, I was stung on the forearm by something. It could have been a stinging caterpillar, but it could also have been a particularly deadly Australian spider, the funnel web. I immediately thought the worst. Especially when I saw the puncture marks on my arm. I rang the Poisons Information Centre.

'Should I go to a hospital?' I panted.

'Not unless you know it was a funnel web that bit you.'

'How will I know?'

'If it was a funnel web, you'll start to feel nauseous in 20–30 minutes. If that happens, get to a hospital. Quickly.'

Can you imagine what I started to feel from that minute on? It turned out not to be a spider bite at all, but for the next 20–30 minutes, every twinge I felt was 'nausea'. Such is the power of suggestion when it comes to health.

Another aspect of Western medicine I find disappointing is that its main healing arm, its nurses, are under increasing pressure to reduce the nurturing that has long been their strength. Invariably this is the outcome of a drive for efficiency in health care, which is another way of saying that society wants cheaper medical services. In my experience, nursing has always been the great hope of orthodox medicine; it forms the bridge between dispassionate science and humanity. It should come as no surprise that nurses have been one of the driving forces in the growing popularity of complementary therapies as adjuncts to mainstream medicine.

So, how significant is the role of the healer?

In any given health situation, there are three factors which can influence the outcome.

The most important is you: your attitudes, your beliefs, and your conviction.

The second most important is the health therapist.

And, possibly, the least important of them all is the therapy itself. You can just about hear the groan of disbelief from the various self-interest groups when they read that: in non-acute situations, the therapy is often the least important part of the healing equation.

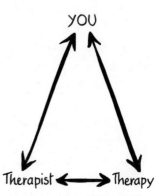

However, all three elements play a role – and they are interlinked. If you play down the importance of one, you usually have to compensate by elevating the role of another. This is a matter of personal choice.

If, for example, you decide that you will accomplish your healing by yourself, with no other support, the requirement from you is increased.

If you decide to hand over all responsibility to a third party (the therapist), then their efforts must, of necessity, be increased.

And if you decide to place all your faith in the therapy alone – whatever it may be – then it has to be one hell of a therapy.

Steps to choosing a health therapist

The first step is to know what you want to achieve. You must believe this is achievable, and you must be wholly committed to it. Then:

- **Research.** Know all there is to know about what you want to achieve, what is entailed and, most important of all, where you want to end up. Seek advice from your primary healthcare provider, support groups, libraries etc.

- **Use the Success Formula** from page 183. Make sure you use the complete Calm Inspiration Cycle as part of this.

- **Ask for referrals**. These can come from medical or alternative practitioners, friends, support groups, colleges, professional associations and healthfood stores.

- **Choose the therapy** or therapies you have most faith in.

- **Interview the therapists.** You are the consumer; you are entitled to interview without obligation. Gauge the level of their commitment. Remember, take notes and trust your instincts.

- Once committed, **have faith** in the therapist and therapy you have chosen – unless your instincts tell you that something is not right. From here on in, it's a healing partnership.

Making all these elements play a role is usually the most expedient solution. So this brings us to the inevitable question: if you are the constant in this equation, and the therapy usually comes as part of the package when you choose a therapist, how on earth do you choose a health therapist?

Should you listen to the therapist who says illness is a choice you make, or the one who says illness chooses you? Should you take notice of the therapist who says you need more exercise, or the one who says you need more rest? Should you listen to the one who says you'll die without chemotherapy, or the one who says chemotherapy will kill you? Or should you, as some people still do, transfer all responsibility to the family doctor?

How are you meant to choose a health therapist?

While you are doing this, it is important to bear in mind the four primary questions that must continually be asked of all therapists, and must be answered to your complete satisfaction before you progress:

(i)   What is the best treatment or therapy for my particular problem?

(ii) What research or evidence exists that proves this is the best treatment or therapy?

(iii) What assurance do I have that this information is reliable?

(iv) What beliefs or emotional requirements must I provide for this treatment or therapy to be effective?

Follow all those steps, do your homework, then follow your instincts. Not your likes or dislikes, your *instincts*.

The role of the therapy

I have already suggested that the therapy is probably the least important element of the healing triumvirate. Many will take exception to that. After billions have been spent on researching a particular disease and its treatment, after exhaustive clinical testing has taken place, surely it is outrageous for a mere author to suggest that the therapy is the least important element in the equation.

In standing by that assertion, I do not question the efficacy of the treatments in question. All I'm suggesting is that *you* play the most important role in this process. If you decide you've had enough of living, the best medical treatment in the world is not going to do you a whole lot of good. Conversely, if you decide you're going to become well, and you'll do anything in your power to achieve this, then even the weakest treatment is strengthened.

Today you have a veritable smorgasbord of therapeutic options to choose from. Orthodox or alternative? Modern or traditional? A doctor–patient relationship or a partnership? Allopathic or homeopathic? Eastern or Western? Psychic or scientific? The choices go on.

And the decisions may be even more complicated than that. Should you submit to surgery right away? Should you wait until you are stronger, using natural remedies and meditation to get you into better shape first? Or should you investigate Chinese medicine instead? Should you use antibiotics or herbal remedies? Chemotherapy or vitamin therapy? Guided imagery or yoga? Anesthetic or acupuncture? Surgery or spiritual healing?

Although having choice is meant to make you feel more at ease, having too many options to choose from can be stressful. So what do you do? How will you know what is the right therapy for you? The only advice I can sincerely offer in these circumstances involves three steps.

- **Meditate** (that is, use Deep Calm) for your health's sake, and until you feel comfortable about exploring one particular direction or another.

- **Investigate**. Take a thorough look at what's on offer, and what you *feel* will work best for you. All therapies work for some people. Few therapies work for all people. Some will work for one type of person, others will work for another. It's personal. Probably the most personal decision you will ever face.

- **Meditate** some more to see whether the therapies you have explored are going to work for you. Listen to your subconscious. The answer is within you.

I can't begin to tell you how often I have been asked for recommendations on treatments and therapies. What is the best? What will work for me? Even a couple of my closest friends have sought this advice from me.

But, as pressured as I feel, and as dearly as I would like to help, I cannot sincerely answer this question for them.

In spite of the successes I know about, and my admiration for many who work in the various fields, I am reluctant to recommend one therapy over another to someone close to me. If you're wondering why, I must remind you of the central theme of this book: when it comes to you and your health, *you* are the expert. There are millions of highly trained medical experts in the world, yet none can equal you when it comes to knowing how you feel and what you require to make yourself well. Not only are you unique in yourself, you are uniquely equipped to make the decisions relating to your wellbeing. If you are to succeed in preserving or restoring your health, you have to take responsibility and make the correct decisions for yourself.

Most people will not feel the urgency to search for an alternative until such time as they believe they have exhausted the possibilities of their current therapy. Then they usually react in one of four ways.

(i)   They abdicate responsibility and hand it over to a third party, such as a specialist.

(ii) They seek alternative cures.

(iii) They try to combine alternative and conventional treatments.

(iv) They do nothing.

My recommendation is that you choose the therapy and therapist you *feel* most comfortable with – ideally before you reach the desperation stage. If you get into the frame of mind where you believe you're struggling for your own survival, you will have to work all the harder to overcome the negative emotions that arise from this.

If your decision is to hand over all responsibility for your health to a third party, only you are in a position to know whether that is the best decision for you. And let us not forget that this is a decision made by millions every day – often with success.

If you decide to pursue alternative therapies, please consider that there is a mainstream when it comes to 'alternatives', and that the popular ones are usually popular for good reason.

The two things I do know about alternatives are that: 'magic bullet' cures you sometimes read about usually have more to do with marketing than they do with healing; and it's unlikely there is a miracle therapy in the jungles of Brazil, the mountains of Rajasthan, or the laboratories of Switzerland that will make the difference in your present situation.

So, with so many choices on offer, where are you supposed to turn?

The role of research

What is the alternative to adhering blindly to a particular approach to healing?

Ignorance is hardly an alternative. After billions have been spent, and some of the world's most brilliant minds have been devoted to discovering what makes you ill and what makes you well, it would be foolhardy to discount this. Even if a prognosis is bleak, knowledge can be more comforting than doubt (for most people). But more importantly, knowledge and understanding may be necessary steps towards finding a solution.

Remember the first step of the complete Calm Inspiration Cycle? The step you undertook before you called on your subconscious to play its role in your decision making? This was the homework, the research, the data-gathering part. Study the topic, gather research, prepare, compare, calculate, evaluate, explore, assess. This is one area that is unforgiving of shortcuts. When your wellbeing is at stake, the last activity you want to skimp on is research.

Know all there is to know about what stands in the way of your wellness. Know what you want to achieve, what it entails, and most important of all, where you want to end up. To do this, you will probably seek advice from your primary healthcare provider; however, you can also get this from support groups, libraries and the Internet – in fact any other source you can think of. I cannot over-emphasise the importance of this research. If there is an expert on your particular condition, seek them out! If there is medical or scientific research on the area that interests you, use it!

Now that I've said that, it's equally important that you understand the potential drawbacks in researching a topic you are technically unable to grasp.

The advantages of research	The disadvantages of research
• You may discover something important in relation to your condition • It may help you to feel more in control • You will feel more capable of making informed decisions • You will have the background information you need for intuitive interpretation	• No matter whom you consult, it is difficult to even get close to the 'big picture' • Statistics are often grossly misleading • It can be an intimidating process • You could cause yourself unnecessary stress

You may choose to explore the Internet for information. Be warned, though, that at a time of fear and uncertainty, you may overlook the fact that there's a lot of unsubstantiated garbage on the Internet. The credentials of web site providers can be hard to establish. More disturbing, once a web page is published, a misleading, poorly researched piece of speculative nonsense can *look* as authoritative as something far more worthy. On the Internet, nihilists get equal prominence with Nobel Prize winners. Pornographers get more prominence than both.

So when you gather information from the Internet you must apply more than your usual level of vigilance, and be prepared to sift through vast amounts of information. Then, at the conclusion of your search, the confusion and contradictions may be insurmountable.

How are you meant to evaluate any one of these therapies, let alone all of them? At the conclusion of this section (page 286) is a technique that will simplify this process.

To review other people's experiences in this area – or to share your own – you will find a special section on this topic at www.calmcentre.com/reader on the Calm Centre's web site; you'll need the password 'reader'.

Before we move on from this section on research, there are three pieces of advice I wish to leave you with.

(i)   The best time to think about your choice of therapy is *before* you need it.

(ii) If you have never heard of a particular therapy before, there may be a very good reason for it.

(iii) If you decide to combine alternative as well as conventional treatments, it is vital that you advise both therapists of your decision.

Finally, if you decide to do nothing, who am I to question your decision? However, if you don't make such a decision, I have an excellent piece of advice for you: make some sort of decision.

The procedure for doing that is the complete Calm Inspiration Cycle (page 225).

The role of belief

Whether you think that you can or that you can't,
you are usually right.

Henry Ford

On the subject of healing, I must tell you about the most successful medical practitioner I have ever met. This person was not a professor, a surgeon or a specialist of any type – she was a general practitioner. She was successful not because she had a state of the art clinic, an understanding nature or a caring bedside manner, but because she had the ability to heal. (Have you ever heard this said about a physician before?) Especially when it came to 'hopeless' cases. Such was her reputation that her waiting list extended for several months, longer than many serious illnesses would tolerate. Nevertheless, her successes grew.

Fascinated by this popularity, I arranged to meet her. And made a remarkable discovery. (I should point out that this took place about 15 years ago when such a way of thinking was indeed remarkable.) To begin with, there were no 10-minute consultations at this surgery. They simply did not happen. All consultations took at least an hour, and during this time she not only listened and examined, but probed as to the nature of the patient's beliefs. You may recognise this as a standard consultative approach to holistic healing, but there was more to her method than this.

Having established what the problem was, and what the client's biases about healing were, she then began to treat them according to what they believed would work. So if her client had great faith in homeopathy, she treated them homeopathically. If the client had more faith in conventional medicine, then she would treat them with drugs or antibiotics. And her methods varied from client to client, according to what they had faith in – diet, vitamins, acupuncture, surgery, herbs, drugs, whatever. In most cases, it did not matter what she believed was the appropriate treatment; it was infinitely more important what *her client* believed.

Because belief plays an essential role in maintaining or re-establishing wellness. Belief is one of the keys to healing. Belief is one of the keys to achievement.

Remember? $(M+B+F)^i = C$

I come across many so-called terminally ill people who have overcome their illnesses by using alternative therapies of one sort or another, some of which I consider bizarre or even ridiculous. But what I think doesn't matter in the slightest; if you believe in a therapy, it can be successful.

This is why chemotherapy works for some people and not for others. This is why herbal treatments work for some people and not for others. No matter what research says, what statistics show, or what other people's experience indicates, if you believe in a certain approach, you can succeed with it.

The role of focus

Twenty-odd years ago, one of my close friends was diagnosed with throat cancer. After visiting all the top specialists, he was advised that it was time for him to go home and tidy up his affairs.

He didn't go home. He went to Manila instead.

And rather than accept the prognosis he had been given, he sought help from a Chinese Chi Kung master he had studied under many years before.

Once again, he committed himself to the disciplines of ancient learning. This time he studied and applied powerful new (old?) skills to effect his own treatment. He dedicated many hours a day to calm, concentration and study of Chi Kung.

By any measure, the effort he applied was extreme. But he believed in it, wholly. And he focused on it, wholly: 3 hours every day for the next 5 years.

Did it cure him? Who knows. All I know is that, today, he is a picture of health – though with a distinctively raspy voice – having mocked his specialists' best predictions for over 20 years. Now, at 70 years of age, he is still achieving the 'impossible' in all aspects of his life; not the least of which is a highly successful series of books on Chi Kung – *The Power of Chi*, *The Power is You* and *Chi – The Power Within*.

All this from the ability to focus and stay calm.

Nowhere is this ability more necessary than when it comes to overcoming illness and regaining sound health. Because at times like this you need to be able to channel all of your energies – physical, emotional and spiritual – into your healing.

In extreme cases, this may mean calling the family together and informing them that they will now be responsible for their own support and sustenance, and that you will be expecting to receive both of these things from them. It may mean quitting your job, so that you can devote your energies to healing; in a life or death situation, this may not be too big a price to pay. This would also mean visiting all your creditors, explaining your situation, and advising them you will not be in a position to keep your payments up to date. If they repossess your house . . . you may conclude that you have something much more important at stake.

Can you see what I'm getting at here? If you are focused on your wellness, rather than other aspects of your life, you may be confronted by difficult decisions – but when all of your energy is focused on healing, you'll be surprised how easy even the 'toughest' decisions will become.

Once again, I know it is easy for me to sit here and write this, while it is much more difficult to put into practice. However, in a life or death situation, you may have to make difficult choices.

Applying the formula

Now we come to the part where we bring all of these elements together in a simple, understandable formula. The purpose of this is to provide direction, answers to questions, suggestions for approaches you should take in your healing efforts.

This is an answer-finding technique. *It is not intended as a healing practice in its own right.*

$$(M+B+F)^i = C$$

C The Consequence is 'wellness'. That is a positive consequence. A negative one would be 'eradicating illness'. You need to create a positive, realistic picture of yourself after having overcome whatever illness or condition is bothering you, and being restored to full health. This will involve either visualisation or a Consequence Montage (page 204). Probably both. You will refer to this healthy, vibrant image often.

M Motivation should be straightforward. Your *positive* motivation is how good it will feel to be vital and well after you have completed this process. Your *negative* motivation, or what will happen if you do not do this, will never be far from your mind.

B Belief is essential. You must find a therapy and a therapist you can believe in. More importantly, you must do whatever it takes to believe in your own ability to achieve the Consequence you have in mind. Carrying around a laminated Consequence Montage in your pocket or handbag will help you achieve that.

F Focus is as we have just described. You must devote all of your energy to the task at hand.

The seven steps to *i*

Now we have to find the most important ingredient, *i*. To do this, we use the complete Calm Inspiration Cycle.

1. Preparation You do your research, gather the information, do your preparation. If it is at all possible, conduct some of this research from a location where you are exposed to new influences (that is, from outside your normal comfort zone); this will challenge your regular thought patterns.

Then define the Consequence you seek. For example: 'What steps should I take to overcome this illness and bring an ongoing sense of wellness and vitality to my life?'

2. Start at the end Imagine yourself having accomplished the Consequence you have defined. Imagine what you'll look like when you are healthy and vital. Imagine looking at your X-rays when they are all clear. Look at the expression of bemusement on your physician's face as he is forced to pronounce, against all his expectations, that you are well again. Do this as thoroughly and as imaginatively as you can manage.

Imagine what you will sound like. Imagine the things you will hear, the things people will say to you, the things you'll say yourself, the note of surprise in the physician's voice. Then imagine how it will feel to hear those things, and to have achieved what you set out to achieve. Imagine how it will feel to be healthy and full of life. Imagine the feeling you will have when your family and friends celebrate the fact that you are well again.

Be creative. Be ambitious. Be as bold as you like – after all, it's only happening in your imagination.

3. Go to the centre Use one of the Step 3 techniques (see pages 145–70) to ease yourself into a state of Deep Calm.

While in this state, don't give another thought to your Consequence. Just enjoy the peace and stillness of Deep Calm, as your body slowly rebuilds its strength and immunity.

4. Accept the answer   At the conclusion of the Deep Calm process, thoughts will come to mind. Whatever they are, however poorly formulated or obscure they may seem, write them down.

This is your subconscious communicating with you.

5. Conscious evaluation   Now it is time to examine what these thoughts mean. This step may be unnecessary if complete thoughts come to mind, or it may be a process that takes several hours. Don't hurry it; this interpretation phase may arouse some of your most creative thinking.

At the conclusion of this, you will have one or more suggestions. Evaluate them. How do these suggestions fit in with what you know (from your research) to be so? Are they practical? Do you feel comfortable with them? Which one do you feel most comfortable with?

If you do not feel comfortable with any, go back to the beginning. Do more research. Look harder. Interrogate your data and information. Be more creative with the brief you give yourself. Then repeat the process.

Remember the answer does *not* have to be logical or rational. It may be intuitive. In extreme cases it may even go against everything you have been told is so – but you still *feel* it is the way to go. This is the way to go.

6. Unconscious evaluation   Assuming a suggestion has passed your conscious evaluation and you have concluded that it has merit, it is time to see whether, deep down, you are convinced by it.

The way you do this is to ease yourself into a deeply relaxed state again, then imagine yourself applying the suggestion your subconscious came up with.

If it feels comfortable, imagine yourself applying this suggestion in other situations.

If it doesn't feel comfortable, then go back to the very first step. More research. More analysis of the available information. A different approach to defining your consequence.

7. Integration   The final stage of the complete Calm Inspiration Cycle is putting it into practice. You have the motivation. By now you will have the belief. Provided you can apply the right degree of focus, you now have that special ingredient, i, which is required to realise your Consequence.

You have the power to heal

I believe that all human beings are capable of accomplishing much more than they have been allowed to believe. Immeasurably more. Usually surpassing their wildest dreams or expectations. Because, in most cases, even their dreams have been constrained. Removing those constraints is what *Calm for Life* is about.

I do not, however, believe in miracles.

I would never suggest to you that all people who follow the healing advice in these pages will achieve, or have achieved, miraculous cures and overcome diagnosed 'terminal' illnesses. In many cases, those illnesses are, or were, indeed terminal. This should not imply failure. If you had been present during the final hours of people who employed the techniques and philosophies from this book, and had asked them whether they had succeeded or failed in their quest, I venture that all would have considered themselves successes. Because sometimes extending life in its present form may not be seen as a desirable goal.

There are always other goals. Part of the challenge is to recognise them.

Having said that, let me concentrate for a moment on those who *did* effect the breakthrough cures and healings, and *did* overcome so-called terminal illnesses. In all cases that I am aware of, two factors were present:

(i)   they learned how to bring peace and calm into their lives;

(ii) they accepted responsibility for their own lives and health, and were determined to play a leading role in the management of both.

When you take responsibility for yourself and for your own state of health, you understand that any treatment or program you undertake will involve all of your being. Even if you hand over responsibility to other parties, complete healing requires your full and uncompromising involvement.

Healing requires more than therapies alone.

Healing requires a close examination of all aspects of your lifestyle, making improvements wherever possible. This will involve a new look at your diet, exercise programs and work responsibilities. This is not optional, it is a necessity.

Healing may also involve detoxification: walking away from those toxins and habits (smoking, drugs and alcohol abuse) that have a negative effect on your health. It may be argued that giving up such habits creates additional stress at a time when you can least accommodate it. This may be so in a few rare cases, but I seriously doubt it. If you 'give up' something, you may very well suffer the stresses of doing so. But what I am proposing is that you 'take up' something more enriching and life-enhancing. If you recall the Calm Centre's Nine Mental Powers, especially the Power of Substitution; you will realise that the most effortless way of overcoming a negative habit or behaviour, is simply to substitute a positive one. Instead of concentrating on giving up smoking, you concentrate on becoming fitter and healthier; instead of concentrating on what you're forgoing (cigarettes), you concentrate on what you're gaining (new diet, new skin-care products, new exercise program, new wardrobe). Because substitution is immeasurably more powerful than will.

Healing will involve living in as clean and healthy an environment as you can manage.

Healing will involve a spring clean of all your emotional baggage. Primarily, this means forgiving everyone who has ever caused you distress – do it for your sake even more than theirs. If you harbour any pain and regret from your past, about your mother, father, past partners or associates, dispense with it. At this very moment, such a suggestion may sound glib, but if your life and future wellbeing is under threat: forgive, forget, move on. Let them worry or harbour grudges if they will – as long as you dispose of yours, with grace, you can move on.

Healing will involve accepting yourself as you are right now, learning to love and appreciate yourself as you are right now. If you have difficulty achieving this, you might want to seek professional guidance. Interview the practitioners. Be aware of what *feels* right. Trust your intuition and don't agree to any extreme practices (that is, what *you* consider to be extreme).

Finally, no matter what else you do, healing should involve extended periods of Deep Calm. In this way, not only will you find it easier to be peaceful and accepting, but you will be on your way to overcoming the fear, resentment and despair that sometimes accompanies serious illness. Extended periods of relaxing Deep Calm will make you feel more positive and in control. And, most important of all, extended periods of Deep Calm will benefit your immune system.

Calm for success and prosperity

Considering that so much of this book has been devoted to a very flexible concept of success, it is appropriate that we explore it in more detail here. Whatever your concept of success, chances are it is something you consider just beyond your reach. Even people that you would consider to be extremely successful are governed by this belief. In other words, success is something to be worked towards, rather than something to be enjoyed at this very moment. It is a quest, or a process, rather than an accomplishment.

When you ask most people to evaluate their lives, in terms of being successful or unsuccessful, they tend to rate themselves poorly. Even when they can list a dozen proud accomplishments in their recent lives, they seldom rate this as successful. It seems few people ever attain the level of success they consider necessary to be able to think of themselves as successful.

When you ask people to evaluate their state of prosperity, you find a similar modesty. There are many that you and I would call wealthy who choose words like 'comfortable' or 'well off' to describe their status. It seems few people ever attain the level of wealth they consider necessary to be able to think of themselves as wealthy. And so it goes.

There are a variety of psychological reasons why people do not achieve or attract the levels of success they desire. Foremost among these are:

- it is not central to their core needs or values;
- they don't think they deserve it;
- they are afraid;
- they don't think they are capable of it;
- they think it's not up to them, and is all a matter of luck, fate or privilege;
- they try too hard.

When you dispense with those reasons, you can concentrate on the main challenge: how success is accomplished.

Your core needs and values

When you have identified your values and priorities, and have structured them as ideals, you have a road map for life. If the Consequences you design for yourself sit neatly on this road map, they are much easier to accomplish.

In no area is this more important than when we are talking about prosperity and success. Most of us would say that such attributes would enrich our lives substantially but, deep down, do we really have that conviction? If not, it's a difficult quest.

So, the first step is simply identifying your values and priorities. That is what the Centenarian Test (page 239) is for. When you do this test, it will probably not highlight the need for wealth and money. Few people identify this as one of their core emotional or spiritual needs.

In spite of this, wealth and money will remain an important consideration all throughout our lives. Why? Some people see wealth as a by-product of success – a measure or a reward. (Others see it as an end product, but that's another story.) More importantly, wealth has the ability to remove one of the most prevalent of life's stressors: financial pressure.

Incidentally, when I refer to wealth, I am not thinking about extreme wealth; I'm talking about the gathering of resources that will enable you to be relaxed and comfortable in life – if that is what you aspire to. The resources needed to do this will vary from person to person. What Bill Gates requires, and what someone who is out of work requires, will probably be quite different.

Do you deserve it?

A few years ago I met a prominent religious personality at the airport in Cleveland, Ohio. Something inside me made me ask what I'm sure most people would secretly want to know: how could he reconcile his quest for wealth with the message he preached?

Without so much as a blush, he explained that money was merely a form of energy. As such, it can flow in a negative direction – to casino operators or bookies – or in a positive direction – to someone who preached hope and goodness, someone not unlike himself.

I'm not sure I approve of his rationalisation, but I was impressed by his uncomplicated attitude towards wealth or success. He felt he was worth it, and therefore would accept it without shame or embarrassment. We often joke about not deserving success, but it is one of the more enduring limitations that people struggle with.

Our lives are governed by beliefs we inherit, learn at home or school, or develop of our own free will for reasons we will never know. More often than not, these beliefs serve to limit, rather than to encourage us. High on the list of limiting beliefs are our attitudes towards wealth, prosperity and achievement. Money is the root of all evil; power corrupts; money can't buy happiness; the rich get richer, the poor get poorer . . . you've heard them all. Yet, while we allow these negative clichés to constrain us, we also subscribe to the belief that wealth and success represents status and freedom.

How do you overcome these contradictions?

Appreciate the fairness The starting point is one very important understanding: whatever good fortune you attract in life, you are not depriving somebody else. No matter how you analyse the universe's resources, there is more than enough food, wealth, love, gratitude and wellness to go round.

Arguments about fairness, railing about the inequity between the 'haves' and the 'have nots', will always exist. But, resisting good fortune does not balance this scale in any way – if anything, it tilts it even further in favour of the 'haves'.

> *Whatever good fortune you attract in life, you are not depriving somebody else.*

Be a magnet Secondly, you will become like a magnet for success if you believe you are a conduit of good fortune to others. Generosity is much more than its own reward: it creates a positive momentum – good fortune comes to you, so that you can help spread it. How wonderful would it be to be in the position when you could give away millions to the less fortunate? How ennobling would it be to know that you have the power to help others?

Prove your worth Many of us have difficulty in accepting our own worth. Is an hour of my time *really* worth that much? Can I *really* expect so much when I have given so little?

One thing in life is sure. You will never be worth more than you think you are worth.

There are two ways to overcome this limiting belief. The first is to readjust your ways of viewing your worth; some people can do that by comparing their contribution with that of others who are successful. The easier way, though, is this: if you doubt the value of your contribution in life, increase your contribution. How easy is that?

Accept graciously When you are grateful for what you have, and for the good fortune that comes your way, it has a habit of continuing to come your way. Don't ask me why – it's just a practice many successful people have told me they employ, and you can't argue with success.

Act successful We have already discussed the power of pretence as a way of convincing the subconscious – *your* subconscious – to adopt certain ways of thinking. It is also an excellent way of calmly overcoming inhibitions about success.

Part of this act is preparing yourself for success. Adopt a successful demeanour. Buy the wardrobe. Learn the acceptance speeches. Allocating the space is particularly useful. 'This is where my assistant will sit (when I get one). Here is where I will entertain my clients (when I attract them).' I know from my own experience that it is a powerful subconscious incentive to success, and it works like a charm!

When you act like a successful person, think like a successful person, mix with successful people and encourage their continued success, and leave room in your life for success to flourish, you just can't fail.

Are you afraid?

To be successful in any field, you have to learn to overcome two irrational, but almost universal, fears: the fear of failure and the fear of success.

Fear of failure is the greatest barrier to success. You see this with people who win a coveted middle-management position, or accumulate a few assets, then cling to these as the measure of their worth. The moment they succumb to that way of thinking they are trapped – too risk-averse to try to raise the stakes, and too comfortable to want to explore new directions. So mediocrity or natural attrition slowly makes its presence felt.

The more you believe you have to lose, the less you have to gain.

One of the observations I've made in business is that it's easier to train someone on a salary of 10,000 to lift their annual income to 500,000, than it is to train someone earning 200,000 to do likewise. Why? Because the latter believes they have more to lose.

When you believe you have much to lose, you act cautiously; the greatest achievements in life always seem to happen when you convince yourself you have nothing to lose. So, unless you can convince yourself to let go of what you have, you will always be constrained by what you have.

You see it happen with relationships. Those who cling to what they have, fighting to preserve it in the form they first discovered it, often lose it altogether. Ironically, this often happens as a result of the relationship going stale because 'nothing ever changes'.

Focus on the adventure and the enriching aspects of growth, as opposed to the negative prospect of losing what you already have, and you must thrive. You can't help but thrive!

The second common fear, which is sometimes even greater than the fear of failure, is the fear of success. What if I do get that job? What if my product really takes off? What if that beautiful man really wants to marry me? Don't scoff, it's one of the most common success inhibitors. And it's closely linked to not wanting to forgo what you already have – even if you are not happy with what you already have.

Now that we have identified the obstacles, overcoming them simply becomes a matter of motivation. And, in searching for this, we have to balance the *negative* motivation of not wanting to risk what you've got against the *positive* motivation of wanting to have something more than you've got.

Which one can you make the stronger?

Creating a positive motivation is a two-step process. The first step involves reducing your negative motivations. The second step involves making your positive motivation so compelling that you simply cannot resist it. I will refer to these motivations almost as if they have personality – which, in a way, they do.

Reducing your negative motivations This is an essential part of the process because negative motivations exist for a good reason. Invariably, their purpose is to protect you from something – failure, pain, embarrassment, loss. And, although you might logically be able to see that they serve no useful purpose (in this particular case), emotionally you will *feel* otherwise.

Negative motivations have to be addressed. And the best way to address them is to replace them with positive ones. (See 'Transposing motivations', opposite.)

Enhancing your positive motivations This is the 'why' part of your equation. Why do you have to succeed? Why is success important to you? How will you feel when you have achieved it? What will it enable you to do?

The more work you put into adding realism to this, to becoming familiar with the feelings associated with it, the easier it becomes to put aside your negative motivations – the forces that hold you back.

Be creative. Add as much colour and interest as you can to this process because that will help you make it more integral.

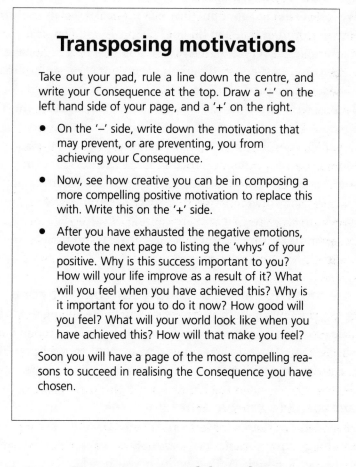

Transposing motivations

Take out your pad, rule a line down the centre, and write your Consequence at the top. Draw a '–' on the left hand side of your page, and a '+' on the right.

- On the '–' side, write down the motivations that may prevent, or are preventing, you from achieving your Consequence.

- Now, see how creative you can be in composing a more compelling positive motivation to replace this with. Write this on the '+' side.

- After you have exhausted the negative emotions, devote the next page to listing the 'whys' of your positive. Why is this success important to you? How will your life improve as a result of it? What will you feel when you have achieved this? Why is it important for you to do it now? How good will you feel? What will your world look like when you have achieved this? How will that make you feel?

Soon you will have a page of the most compelling reasons to succeed in realising the Consequence you have chosen.

Are you capable of it?

This is the telling moment for many of us once we have designed an ambitious Consequence for ourselves. Can we pull it off?

It's easy for some semi-reclusive author to say you can dream the big dreams, then go chasing them, but what if you're trapped in a house with four kids under 10? What if you've been unemployed for the past 3 years? What if you've injured your back and can't work without pain?

These are things that only you can answer. And, if you prepare yourself effectively, these answers will come to you when you ease yourself into your most creative state – Deep Calm. In this state, you will be aware of your potential.

We're not talking about pulling fantasies out of the air that are not important to you or that you do not believe, deep down, that you will ever accomplish. Everyone can say, 'I'm going to be a billionaire', but not everyone can do it. Everyone can say, 'I'm going to win Wimbledon next year', but not everyone can do it.

This is why you formulate your Consequence using the Calm Inspiration Cycle. So that all your creativity and inspiration will reveal what is possible for you – as well as how it can be made possible. This is a subconscious process that evaluates all your known resources in a way that you cannot do consciously. Then, by applying the various steps elements of the Success Formula, you can consciously convince yourself you are capable of it.

In addition to this, however, I have two recommendations that will extend your capacities immeasurably:

Be prepared to move beyond your comfort zone Your comfort zone is what binds you to what you know and presently have; because of this, it is also what holds you back. Pushing these comfort boundaries from time to time opens your mind to new possibilities and acquaints you with the possibility of going much further.

Be prepared to receive what you seek This sounds obvious, but is widely overlooked. Many people are bold enough to ask for extraordinary things in life, but that is as far as they take it. Asking is nowhere near enough. Asking will get you nowhere . . . unless you are open to receiving.

Years ago, when I was a business consultant, I noticed how companies that were focused on growth and expansion through attracting new business invariably attracted new business. Almost without exception. Perhaps you see nothing unusual about this, except that, in the majority of cases, the business they attracted did not come from the areas they were concentrating on – it came from totally unexpected places. Even when they had highly disciplined, structured new business programs, the opportunities frequently came from unexplored areas. Conversely, companies who were not focused on growth or expansion programs, even though they were desperate for additional business, enjoyed few of these unexpected 'coincidences'.

While management consultants may frown on the unpredictability of this practice, successful entrepreneurs are very aware of it, and try to capitalise on it. You know what I think it is? Simply being open to success. Being prepared to accept whatever you seek.

Try this: walk to your front door right now. Open it. Stand there for a moment, looking out at the world. Now, extend your arms as wide as possible, throw your head back, and say very clearly to yourself: 'I'm ready'.

The more often you do this, the sooner you will be ready.

What about luck?

'It's out of my hands,' she said. 'I've never been a lucky person.'

Have you ever noticed how misfortune often seems to focus more on the unfortunate and downtrodden than on those you classify as successful? And have you ever noticed how successful businesses and people always seem to attract even more (often unrelated) good fortune than the struggling ones?

Is this luck?

Have you ever watched a football game and noticed how often a fluke breeze or the bounce of the ball seem to favour the really hot team? Whether they win or lose, the hot team usually gets all the breaks. It happens time after time. Sporting commentators have a cliché for this: 'Good players make their own luck'.

Luck?

It is no secret that one of the greatest injustices of life is that good luck usually favours those who seem to have plenty of it, while bad luck befalls those who are least equipped to deal with it. Pessimists become accident-prone. Depressed people find depressing things happening to them. Unhappy people are burdened by more and more unhappiness. 'Bad luck comes in threes'. Are you getting some sort of picture here?

Popular wisdom tells us that the opposite also applies. Optimistic people attract 'luck', as do positive people, highly focused people, motivated people, and those who know where they're going in life. When you know where you're heading, and concentrate on the path, good fortune has a habit of coming along with you.

Do you try too hard?

One of the great paradoxes in life is that in the physical world, more effort produces greater results while, in the mental world, *less* effort produces greater results.

Nowhere is this more evident that when you're pursuing success.

Just as the martial artist is severely weakened when he is tense or anxious, so too is the business executive, the salesperson, the new parent, or the chef. All of these people are at their most capable when they are centred, with a state of inner calm.

Relax. Success comes much more easily than you think.

How do you do it?

Once all the other elements are in place, finding the way to creating your success is the easy part. All you have to do is follow the formula.

$$(M+B+F)^i = C$$

The Consequence is whatever you choose to pursue for yourself.

Your Motivation is how good it will feel to have achieved your goal, and how bad it will feel if you fail to do so.

Your Belief is that you deserve success, and are capable of it.

Your Focus is on this quest, to the exclusion of almost all else in life.

The inspired element, i, shows you how to achieve all of this. You determine this by carrying out the steps in the Calm Inspiration Cycle.

Relax. Success and prosperity are much closer than you think.

Calm and be happy

Parts of the past 15 years have been pretty depressing. I've attended and participated in countless lectures and talk shows, trying to appear knowledgeable about conditions like stress, anxiety and depression.

Many of these discussions centred around the notion that these are illnesses or medical conditions. Fortunately, according to this perception, there is always a new 'wonder drug' that will solve the problem. (I can remember a time when valium was considered the wonder drug.) Yet, in spite of all these wonderful drugs, futurists tell us that the most significant medical problem we're going to have to face over the next 20–30 years is not starvation, but depression.

Bleak, isn't it?

It would take a daring person to suggest that many of these ailments sound less like physiological ailments – as they are so often treated – and more like ailments of the spirit. But are you prepared to consider that possibility for a moment?

- Are you prepared to consider that an overall state of unhappiness or dissatisfaction may be more debilitating than all the neuro-chemical, hormonal or genetic imbalances combined?

- Are you prepared to concede that many of the psychological and physiological aberrations that accompany these conditions may be the *effects* of the condition rather than the cause?

- Are you prepared to consider the possibility that a simple change of physiology can, in many cases, transform the way someone feels about their life?

- Are you prepared to consider that many mood disorders are the product of nutritional deficiencies, and that people who are inclined towards these disorders may require more than the usual amounts of vitamins, minerals and amino acids?

You should.

Because if only some of these possibilities are true, think how much control you can have over how you're going to feel in the future.

Are you happy now?

A couple of years ago my assistant came hurrying into work, excitedly going on about a show she'd seen on television the previous evening – a BBC program about a bold experiment that had taken place in Oxford, England, the year before.

'It was called something like the Happiness Project. You'd love what they were doing. It fits perfectly with what we're doing. We have to make contact.'

My enthusiasm was no match for hers. This was understandable: it was early in the morning and I was preparing for my first meeting of the day. It was to be with a man who'd set up an appointment via email months earlier. He'd flown out from England. His name was Ben Renshaw.

It did not take long for him to get to the point of the meeting. He had been working on a project with a man called Robert Holden. Within minutes, he had newspaper clippings about this project spread all over my table. One of these in particular stood out. 'The Happiness Project.'

The Happiness Project? Where had I heard of that before?

At that moment my assistant walked in, saw the clipping, then bounded around the table excitedly. This was the project she had been telling me about! Just a few minutes earlier! The one she'd seen on television. The Happiness Project.

Following a 'coincidence' like that, what would you do? I flew to Oxford to meet with Robert Holden, the director of the Happiness Project. Ever since, I have carried a deep affection for his work.

Central to Holden's happiness message is the understanding that happiness is not an objective. It is a process. All those people working towards happiness, or striving for happiness, are actually denying themselves the pleasure of the experience right now.

How many people do you know who have come to the conclusion that they will only be happy when they have a house in the country, reach the top of their profession, meet the perfect man, drive a Porsche or fit into a size 12 dress?

Then, after they've got their house in the country, or reached the top of their profession, or fit into a size 12 dress, they make a remarkable discovery: they're still unhappy. Because if you can't be happy where you are now, you probably won't be any happier if you move on to somewhere else.

So be happy now.

Happiness is not a result. It is a decision.

To quote Holden's book, *Happiness Now,* 'Time cannot make you happy; attitude can. It is a way of travelling, not a destination'.

Make the decision to be happy. You can be. Right now. All you have to do is make the decision – and think about it.

Start your future now

Maybe you can see obstacles that prevent you from believing you can be happy. Whether these obstacles have substance or not, if you *believe* they have substance, they can prevent you from achieving what you'd like to achieve.

If you do feel that way, nothing I can say will convince you otherwise; your objections will probably be deeply rooted. But you can overcome them! Here is a way you can sidestep almost all of those obstacles and move straight on to happiness now.

Truly, this is not such a big deal. You just *think* it's a big deal.

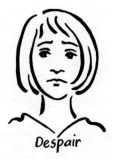

Despair

The difference between the depths of despair and feeling on top of the world is nothing more than the activity of a tiny electrical circuit in your brain.

It is known as a neural pathway, and you can modify it with the most subtle shift of consciousness.

Here are two simple ways you can do it.

The first of these ways is the core of the Calm Inspiration Cycle. Remember the three stages of effecting positive change in your life?

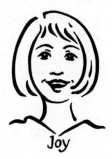

Joy

- Start at the end

- Go to the centre

- Accept the answer

You can use this formula to bring happiness into your life now.

Start at the end   Relax. Tell yourself you have all the time in the world. There was a time, somewhere in your past, when you were happy. Wonderfully, contentedly, peacefully happy.

Maybe you were a child. Or had just got married. Or you witnessed a cloud parting to flood sunlight over the most magical valley you have ever seen. Think back.

Recall that time. Think about it in detail. Great detail. How did you look? What were you wearing? How did you sound? What other sounds did you hear? *What did you feel?* Indulge yourself in this recollection for a few minutes. Go on, immerse yourself in it.

That feeling you are experiencing is the one you want to reproduce. For want of a better word, let's call it happiness.

You were smiling, right? Are you smiling now?

Now that you know what the experience *feels* like, ask yourself the question, 'What do I have to do to be able to feel happiness and joy now? What do I have to do to experience real happiness – at this instant?'

That is your brief.

Go to the centre   You will be getting very familiar with this approach by now. Going to your calm centre. Experiencing Deep Calm. Ignoring the issue you are concerned with, and simply enjoying the pleasure of calm. Having all the time in the world at your disposal.

Think only about becoming relaxed, moving into a deeper state of relaxation. The happiness issue will be the farthermost thing from your mind.

Accept the answer   In this instance, the answer you get may not be something you will consciously understand. Possibly it will be something very subtle and internal. Intuitively, you will know whether you have it.

Accept this answer. And trust in your subconscious to help bring it to reality. Happiness can be as accessible as that.

An alternative approach is even easier – and is guaranteed to work in only 15 minutes. It's called the Happy Pretence.

The Happy Pretence

Go somewhere quiet, just relax, and tell yourself you have all the time in the world.

- Think back to a time when you were happy. Wonderfully, contentedly, peacefully happy. Think about it in detail. How did you look? What were you wearing? How did you sound? What other sounds did you hear? *What did you feel?*

- Imagine yourself being like that now. Happy, contented, peaceful.

- Now, start pretending you are exactly like the person you are imagining. Act as if you really were as happy as that. Be as lavish as you like in your pretence – no-one will notice, only your subconscious.

- Remember it's important to speak as if you really were feeling as happy as you're pretending to feel. Use the words that relate to that happy state.

- Next, pretend that others see you as the happy, calm person you're pretending to be.

Can you imagine anything easier than that?

Just pretend you're happy, and you'll be happy. Pretend often enough, and you'll forge new 'happy' neural pathways in your brain that will allow you to see the world in a bold new light.

Calm relationships

Most relationship problems are fuelled by tension. Arguments, fights, jealousies, misunderstandings and, most common of all, expectations not being met. You would think, then, that being able to maintain a semblance of calm and peace in a relationship would not only be an enhancement, but would be almost blissful.

I work with a number of people who specialise in the field of relationship counselling. Invariably, they are intrigued by the possibility of bringing calm to relationships and thus increasing the harmony, improving communications and lifting the overall comfort level of the relationship. The question they most often ask of me is, 'Does being calm enhance relationships?'

Asking an author about relationships is a little like asking a prisoner about life on the other side. Since most authors are, by professional necessity, reclusive creatures who spend long hours locked in messy rooms, obsessively picking over dusty volumes and the hidden little crevices in their brains, they are not usually considered great role models for relationships. So I asked my wife whether being calm enhances relationships. She laughed, and has still not ventured an opinion. My children, however, think it could be enriching.

But relationships involve much more than families and partners. There are relationships in all facets of your life – with your workmates, greengrocer, boss, hairdresser, garage attendant, clients, indeed everyone you come into contact with each day. There are an infinite number of factors that can enrich, impede, confuse, complicate and damage your relationships with them.

Being able to approach such relationships from a perspective of personal calm is a powerful asset. Why? It's a question of dynamics: when your starting point is a state of inner calm, it is a simple matter to add the tension and excitement if you need it; but if your starting point is a state of tension, you have no room to move. (This is one of the principles of martial arts; but that's another story.) So, in a practical sense, how can you bring calm to your relationships?

Obviously the starting point is knowing how to bring calm to yourself. If you are calm, it follows that your relationships will be calmer. Assuming that you have absorbed some of the techniques covered earlier in this book, I have a superb little calming method which helps to spread calm to those around you.

Adding calm

Have you ever been in a roomful of relaxed people when a stress-merchant bursts in – speaking quickly, acting aggressively – and the next thing you know you have a room full of tense people?

You've seen it happen a hundred times. A tense person spreads tension in no time at all.

Fortunately, the converse is also true. A calm person spreads calm.

You've probably had this experience as well. A roomful of anxious people, worried, tense, frowning. Then in floats someone who is absolutely calm and at peace. And, before you know it, the whole room has begun to ease down and become relaxed.

Because just as a tense person spreads tension, a calm person spreads calm.

Calming the room

Anywhere you go where people are tense, you can calm them down – at least a little – by adopting the characteristics of a calm person.

- Purposely slow down your movements, just a little slower than you think would appear normal.

- Then purposely slow down your breathing. (This may not be consciously noticed by the other people but, subconsciously, it will make the point strongly.)

- Next, slow down your speech until it sounds just a little slower than you think is normal.

Before you know it, two things will have happened. You will be calm yourself. And everyone else will have calmed down as well.

Knowing this can place you in a very powerful position. Simply by appearing to be a perfectly calm person, you can encourage others to become calm. You don't even have to be calm yourself; all you need are the outward manifestations of calm. In other words, you can pretend to be calm and still have the same calming effect.

Are you beginning to see the possibilities of this skill?

This works in almost all situations. Whether you are with one person or ten. The only time it may not work is in situations of confrontation – where it may tend to aggravate things. But even in this situation knowing how to remain calm can help. Just ensure your transition into your 'calm mode' is not too sudden; calm down gradually, make sure others are paying attention, and everyone will start to follow.

This is a rapport-building process that uses the natural inclination of tense people to want to slow down. Employing this technique can bring calm to your relationships, but how much of an enhancement this is, only you can judge.

Adding understanding

What I believe is the greatest enhancement to any relationship is not the level of calm, but the level of understanding. After all, relationships live and die on the strength of communication.

As we have already explored, there are as many realities in the universe as there are people. Psychologically speaking, each person is a product of millions of events, experiences and prejudices – most of which they will never understand or even be aware of. So when you try to harmonise these individual 'realities' in a relationship of two or more people, the variables are infinite. These variables make it impossible to be too prescriptive about what sort of procedures will improve communication.

So how can your communication be enhanced to overcome these human limitations? How can you add understanding?

When most people speak of communication or understanding, they will be thinking of words and intent: 'I want to understand, therefore I will understand.' Or the converse: 'I will speak openly about my needs and feelings, therefore the other person will understand.'

Unfortunately, something often stands in the way of this procedure. Words.

You know from experience that in many situations, no matter how much effort you invest in trying to convey your innermost feelings or impressions, your words always seem to be misunderstood. Even though you've weighed up each word, considered all possible misreadings and chosen the most straightforward phrases to articulate your thoughts, you still can't get your point across.

Why? Because we place so much emphasis and reliance on words. Yet, no matter how you choose them or combine them, words account for only a fraction of what your communications convey; in fact, they have a habit of getting in the way of understanding. Communication experts estimate that, in any given situation, words account for no more than ten percent of the meaning imparted. That means ninety percent of the impression you're conveying is coming from factors other than words. Imagine how *that* could further complicate your efforts at communication!

It is interesting to compare the brain scans of people in conversation. Frequently, you find one person with elevated beta-intense brainwaves speaking to another person with elevated alpha-relaxed and theta-open brainwaves. You could ascertain from this that person A is conversing from a more conscious or left-brain perspective (logical, linear and words-orientated), while person B is conversing from a more subconscious or right-brain standpoint (emotional and intuitive).

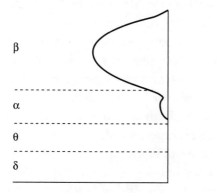

Person A's brainwaves

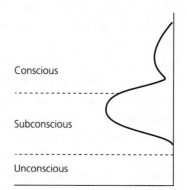

Person B's brainwaves

So person A is relying on the meaning of their words, while person B is responding to subtleties in tone and body language. No wonder there is often so much disparity in communication.

When it comes to the way you communicate with others, you can improve things – to an extent – by relying less on what you say and more on what you feel. However, when it comes to *understanding* somebody else's efforts at communication, you significantly improve the odds if you do just one thing: go to your calm centre – that deeply relaxed place within you – then listen and observe . . . *from inside*.

Widen your peripheral vision (page 133), and allow your tongue to relax, as if it were floating inside your mouth (page 135). These two activities elevate your alpha-relaxed brainwaves, and tend to de-emphasise your analytical processes. In doing this, you will absorb more of the other person's intent, and be less affected by the words themselves. (Many psychotherapists work this way when listening for the meaning behind the words.) However, lest you be seen as glazed-eyed or uninterested, it is important to add one more dimension to this – try to reflect the physiology of the person who is speaking to you: if they're relaxed and laid back, then you should be relaxed and laid back; if they're tense and leaning forward, then you should be tense and leaning forward. Likewise, you should emulate the pace of their words, the rate of their breathing, and the way they sit or stand. If you do this subtly, you will build rapport.

However, empathy and real understanding happens at a much deeper level. Intuitive, unconscious understanding between people involves an additional brainwave activity, one which occurs at the delta level, the level you normally associate with sleep. When they are present during normal waking states, delta-zzz waves facilitate intuition, synchronistic behaviour and psychic communication. Therefore, if two people experience similar levels of delta-zzz waves while they are trying to communicate, both would understand one another with a clarity that is not often experienced.

I can recall hundreds of occurrences of this nature in my relationships, but probably none so pronounced as one that took place in my youth. I was travelling from London to the Isle of Wight for Bob Dylan's comeback concert in the early 1970s. For the duration of the long, lazy train ride I had been making polite small talk with an attractive woman beside me. It was shy conversation about nothing in particular; and certainly bore no relation to the thoughts that were going through my mind about her – thoughts which I was far too reserved to ever let show.

Then, out of the blue, she said: 'Don't think that unless you mean it.' She was as embarrassed by her outburst as I was. The subject we had been discussing was totally unrelated to her comment, yet both of us were immediately aware of its relevance. The real communication had been taking place at an intuitive level, and was only brought into the conscious realm by her impromptu warning.

You will have encountered many communications of similar subtlety in your relationships with others. When it happens, you may try to dismiss the feeling, usually by analysing it until it no longer seems reasonable; you do this in the belief that what you see and hear is more dependable than what you *feel*. But how often do you discover that this is simply not the case?

When two people's delta-zzz brainwaves are elevated, understanding can be greatly enhanced. This is why the purest form of communication takes place when a mother breastfeeds a baby – brainwave scans of mother and baby often reveal inordinately high, and comparable, levels of delta-zzz brainwaves. Similarly, when a couple make love, slowly and calmly, there will be a synchrony in the intensity of their delta-zzz levels, and their communication potential will be at its most profound.

Knowing this, however, may not make it easier for you. Because, unlike alpha, beta and perhaps even theta brainwaves, you cannot consciously turn on delta activity on a whim. However, there are times when delta brainwaves are enhanced:

- when you're deeply relaxed;

- when you indulge in deep and loving thoughts;

- when you engage in quiet, reflective activities;

- when you experience loving, intimate physical contact;

- when you use centring techniques, such as Visiting the centre (see page 144).

At these times, the less stimulation, the fewer thoughts and judgements, the greater will be the understanding. (You will recall the Power of Calm from the Calm Centre's Nine Mental Powers: in matters of the mind, the more mental effort you apply, the less will be the result.)

Please bear in mind that the above relates to your understanding; if you want to ensure the other party understands your communication, it helps if they're in a similar state to you. And that brings us back to the considerations about adding calm, or spreading calm, at the beginning of this section.

Adding reciprocity

Communication is a two-way process: for it to exist, there must be a giver and a recipient: if one gives and the other fails to receive, there is no communication.

You will be aware of the law of reciprocity, where you only get back what you give out. Nowhere is this more true than in the area of love and relationships. If your starting point is to expect love, or to demand love, you will find it seldom materialises; think back on the times in your life when you had expectations of this sort – how often did they end in frustration? To give, without expectation, always attracts the greatest rewards. When you spread loving thoughts, you will attract love in return.

However, it would be overly romantic of us to pretend there aren't occasions in relationships when our focus is not on giving, but on what we get out of these relationships. At times such as this, there is a formula you can apply that will allow you to realise what you want to achieve. You guessed it, it's the core Calm Inspiration Cycle once again: Start at the end; Go to the centre; Accept the answer.

A calm change of habit

We live in an era that is being defined by change. It appears to be the one constant in our lives. Moreover, we've been warned by futurists that this change is exponential, that we haven't even begun to experience what it's really going to be like.

Is that good?

Most people think not. Even those thrill-seekers who profess to enjoy the stimulating possibilities of change tend to have changes of mind when they see something precious to them being threatened. So it's quite natural to feel a little apprehensive about all the change that's taking place in the world.

But, just for a moment, let's examine what change means to you.

Answer this honestly: are you totally happy with the way your life is at this moment? Is your position at work as good as you would ever want it to be? Is your income as reliable and bountiful as you would like it to be? Is your relationship, if you have one, as satisfying as it could possibly be? Is your health, or state of fitness, or attitudes, or lifestyle, as good as you can imagine them being?

Nine times out of ten, your answer to those questions will be, 'Yes, it is possible for these things to be improved on'.

There! You have a vested interest in change.

If you look closely, you will find this exists in all aspects of your life. Sometimes you will even crave change.

'If I ever eat that same meal again, I'll scream.'

'I want to go somewhere different for my vacation this year. What about Venice?'

'If she mentions her aches and pains to me again, I'll tell her what I think.'

Usually, the most desirable area of change will be when it's to do with your own habits, behaviours or attitudes. You can easily change these.

The difference between being a slave to habit and being free and in control is, in most cases, nothing more than the activity of a tiny electrical circuit in your brain. A neural pathway. You can modify it with the most subtle shift of consciousness.

How can knowing how to use Deep Calm help you to effect these changes? Is it possible to use it to achieve things like giving up smoking, losing weight, overcoming stress, cutting down on your drinking?

It is. But first, we must put your objectives into a format that you will find easy to implement.

In Chapter 7 we discovered a method of turning a wish or ambition into a powerful Consequence – one that you can easily work towards turning into a reality. To make it real, your Consequence must be specific, holistic, positive and present. For example, 'I am on the way to becoming a healthy, vital non-smoker. I am on the way to having spotless lungs with boundless capacity.'

Now you have a powerful Consequence! To make it even more real and more powerful, you can create a Consequence Montage (see page 204) that you can refer to several times a day.

And, once you have a well-established Consequence in mind, it becomes a simple matter of applying the Success Formula from page 183:

$$\left(M+B+F\right)^{i}=C$$

Habits, attitudes, behaviours and obsessions are difficult to remove, but easy to replace – as you will recall from the Power of Substitution (page 100). The reasons habits and behaviours exist are not always easy to understand; nor are they *necessary* to understand. But they exist for reasons that your subconscious or unconscious find significant; therefore, you must replace them with more positive habits or behaviours that your subconscious will also find significant.

As long as you approach this from a calm perspective, using Deep Calm practices often, you will identify the positive habits or behaviours that are most significant, and that will be most beneficial for you.

The spiritual side to calm

Science without religion is lame. Religion without science is blind.

Albert Einstein

If there is one element that has shaped the history of mankind more than any other, it is the pursuit of spiritual meaning or fulfilment.

Why?

Is there an instinctive knowledge within us that compels us to think this way? Is it due to the brain's so-called 'God Spot', which seems to be associated with feelings of transcendence? Is it learned? Does it matter? Or is it, as the sceptics say, all based on ignorance?

One of the primary human drives is curiosity, the search for meaning. Throughout history, therefore, spirituality and religion have played a dominant role in attempting to satisfy this need. For as long as there have been records of human activity, there seems to have been a preoccupation with the sacred or the divine.

There is a theory that most, if not all, the world religions stem from actual experiences – either transcendental or metaphysical. With no other way of explaining these, they were described as experiences of the divine. Curiously, this concept of 'divine' did not begin as an attempt to rationalise God, but as a way of trying to rationalise the experience. These rationalisations became ever more complex with the passage of time, the inclusion of new experiences, and the expansion of geographical boundaries and followers.

The important point is that the origins of spiritual development are probably based on experience rather than revelation. (I apologise if that conflicts with your religious beliefs. I'll make it up to you as the chapter progresses.)

In recent years, the quest for a spiritual experience, particularly transcendental experience, has grown to the extent that it has become a potent new force in spiritual development – as it used to be in most of the Western religions, and still is in the East. Whereas, for the past few hundred years, we have been content to treat spirituality as a structured, cerebral activity, we are now beginning to demand the actual experience once again.

You might wonder what is driving this change. Is it simply frustration with the way of the world? Is it part of the never-ending search for transcendence or enlightenment? Or is it a quest for direction in an age defined by a lack of leadership?

It's probably a combination of all of those – all of which are addressed by the three means of acquiring spiritual insight: transcendence, enlightenment and revelation.

Transcendence Transcendence literally means beyond the grasp of normal human reason, description, experience or belief. Transcendence is when you surpass human experience, or when you are no longer limited by the material universe.

While transcendental experience is sometimes the goal of those seeking some sort of mystical high, it is also thought to be the most common form of spiritual *feeling* (an inadequate word, but you will get my meaning). It begins with a glimpse, or hunch, or conceptualisation of something beyond our normal sensory awareness and even our capacity to comprehend.

This could relate to many experiences. Transcendence can come from standing at the top of a mountain, looking out over an unspoiled valley below. It can come from a majestic symphony, when the sounds of all the instruments meld for one glorious moment and transport you to 'another place'. It can happen thirty metres underwater when you look up and see a pair of dolphins frolicking in the diffuse light above you. It can happen at the birth of a baby. And it happens in Deep Calm.

What turns transcendence into a spiritual experience is when you feel in some way connected with what lies beyond. It is not essential that you can identify the source of your transcendent feelings – God, self, the universe, nature, the planets, dolphins, aliens – only that the feelings exist. And, once that connection is made, there is the conviction that you are spiritually, and possibly even physically, part of this source: intrinsic, inseparable and infinite.

That is transcendence.

Enlightenment You know what enlightenment means. Most people think about it as being a breakthrough in understanding, as in: 'Ah, now I get it!'

For centuries, spiritually orientated people have professed a longing for enlightenment. Or at least they've paid lip-service to this ideal. Generally, it is considered to be the product of a lifetime (more or less) struggle for meaning and understanding. In this context, it belongs to the 'no pain, no gain' school of philosophy.

The Western approach tends to be intellectual and didactic. Adherents believe they can become enlightened through a rationalised, educative process, poring over endless written volumes, studying scriptures of various types. I wonder what degree of enlightenment can be taught or learned this way.

In many Eastern spiritual traditions, the path to enlightenment is strewn with obfuscation, requiring years of dedicated service – usually without explanation of its purpose. Possibly, the purpose of this is to exhaust rational curiosity and thus open up another less conscious level of understanding – but this has never been confirmed to me.

In a spiritual context, enlightenment is nothing more than pure awareness: where all thought is suspended, where time and space do not exist, and where you are simply aware of awareness. It is at this moment that you realise your entire existence is nothing more than awareness itself. There is a profound sense of peace, oneness, safety and freedom that accompanies this realisation.

Those who profess to having experienced it report being awash with the pure experience of being. But they also report that the piercing clarity of understanding that accompanies this state does not come as a surprise – it is profoundly familiar and comfortable.

And here we are confronted by the same paradox that appears in the second of the Nine Mental Powers, the Power of Calm: understanding grows as your thinking decreases. The less you think, the less stimuli you respond to, the greater your understanding.

Some Eastern descriptions of this absence of thought and stimuli refer to it as 'the void'. That word may have negative connotations for you, but once you have been there and experienced it for yourself, you will see the wonder of this 'place', and the attraction of it. Indeed, this is the experience that most meditators have had at one time or another, and strive to recapture.

Once you experience pure awareness on your path to enlightenment, the next step is self-realisation: when you become aware of yourself as an eternal being, or become aware of your own eternal awareness.

Revelation   Most religious teaching is based on revelation. 'Someone revealed this to me; now I can share it with you.' Even though this appears to run counter to transcendental experience, revelation is the most acceptably human approach to spirituality.

The ascetic fasts for weeks on end, taking only water and green tea. He meditates for long hours every day. He denies himself all human comfort. Then, in a state of semi-deprivation, he sees the archangel. A revelation.

The leader of the cult presses on the closed eyes of his under-nourished, sleep-deprived disciple. This pressure creates the impression of light and movement – and, through closed eyes, in a religious ecstasy, another young man discovers the truth. Yet another revelation.

A troubled soul comes from the back row of the congregation; she goes up to the stage; a hand is placed on her forehead, an expulsion of breath, a gasp and . . . 'You're saved, sister!' And, sure enough, the revelation is both real and transforming for her.

Some say that revelation is necessary only for those who are not open to spiritual awakening. They compare it to walking around with your eyes closed, suddenly opening them, and crying out that now you can see.

In addition, all over the world, revelatory transformations are taking place without any pretence of spirituality. These are changing the lives of attendees of self-transformation courses – marathons of introspection and dream-building, where you cast off the shackles and hang-ups of your past to embrace a glittering new future. Revelation. Transformation.

A leap of faith

There is another way to spiritual knowledge – and possibly spiritual insight – which is the most common of all.

It is the substance of almost all religions. Nineteenth-century philosopher Søren Kierkegaard called it the 'leap of faith', the mechanism that describes someone's commitment to an objective uncertainty such as God, usually at the instigation of a teacher of some kind. Assuming that God or the hereafter cannot be explained by rational argument and objective proof, the only way to bridge this gap in human understanding is through a leap of faith.

This is not as radical as it appears. For most people, a similar leap of faith is required to accept the existence of an atom, or a light year, or a brain cell. I suspect a leap of faith is more psychological than spiritual – though millions would say that spiritual development comes as a result of making the leap. In other words, make the commitment and spiritual development follows.

If spiritual insight follows from this, it probably still does so through transcendence, enlightenment or revelation.

Who has the answers?

Spiritual awareness. Is it important? Can it exist without religious doctrine? Is the world better as a result of it? Is it something that must be explained rather than sensed? Is one form superior to another? Does it depend on truth and revelation? Can it exist without transcendence? Is its ultimate purpose enlightenment? Is it a necessary part of evolution? Is it instinctive or learned?

It is human nature to want someone else to provide all the answers. But as we have been discovering all the way through this book, there can be an infinite number of answers to any given question, and there is no one answer that can be correct for all people.

This particularly applies to questions of a spiritual nature. The answer that is right for you may not be right for a person in Cambodia or Angola, whether or not you or I believe this answer to be the truth. You know from your own experience that six people from your street or workplace will have six contrasting answers on what is spiritually correct. Does this mean five will be wrong?

A few years back, the London *Times* printed an article referring to me as the 'guru of calm'. It was probably intended as a tongue-in-cheek reference, but not everyone read it that way. For months I received requests from people seeking philosophical input on a variety of questions relating to life's meaning (assisted by the fact that I include my email address in the back of my books).

At first I did what any non-guru would do, and said, 'The meaning of life? I'll get back to you'. But after a few months of this, it dawned on me that there was in fact a very simple answer to this question. According to my perspective – and I apologise if this clashes with your religious sensibilities – the answer is that there is a good probability that there is no meaning to life. At least, no *inherent* meaning to life.

You create your own meaning. You give meaning to your own life.

You can choose to accept this responsibility or hand it over to someone else. Even if you believe your life is dictated by other people or events, you can still be in the driver's seat – if you choose to be. Make this choice and life can be as modern scientists and ancient philosophers alike have been insisting: we create our own worlds, our own universes. In this context, the thought that 'I am the Creator', or that 'God is within me' may be neither pompous nor extreme. Of course, if you follow Buddhist or Taoist traditions, you will not think it in the least extreme.

On the other hand, if you subscribe to the belief that the world was created by an omnipotent Being, then life probably *does* have an inherent meaning (assuming it was created with a purpose). But that still brings me back to my original point: as far as your life is concerned, you can create your own meaning.

What an opportunity!

Imagine how liberated you will feel when you discover that others – parents, partners, teachers, governments, the multinationals, media, extraterrestrials – are no longer responsible for the meaning you take from life. And that just by employing certain strategies and techniques, you can vary this meaning to suit your needs or wishes. Wouldn't this present you with an inspiring array of choices?

It does not require money, power, position, education or special training to do this, as it all takes place within the confines of your mind. You're going to love how easy it is to accomplish.

From calm comes meaning

If you have ever experienced a moment of absolute calm, where your thoughts are stilled, and you are aware of nothing but your own awareness, one of two things will happen. Either you will suddenly become aware of the uniqueness of your state – whereupon your thoughts resume and the state vanishes as if it were never there . . . or you will simply 'be'. As far as I know, there is no midway point. It's one or the other.

The ideal, naturally enough, is the second. This is the aim of all meditation techniques – to focus your attention on 'being' rather than 'doing'.

What follows is my attempt to describe the indescribable: the experience of Deep Calm as it relates to spiritual development. I'm afraid everyday language is a little limiting in this respect: it is difficult to find precise descriptions for what is essentially a transcendental experience. (Meditation and spiritual gurus get around this by using fuzzy mystical metaphors which can be interpreted in any number of ways by the people who hear them. I find this even more imprecise.)

I urge you to read what follows with a clear, open mind. Let your peripheral vision widen as you take in these words. When it comes, allow the bigger picture to formulate without concentrating too hard on these words. (I think you will get the picture.)

As you enter into the state of Deep Calm, there will be three aspects to your experience.

Centred When you are in the Deep Calm state, your attention is totally centred. You will be conscious of this. From a clear point within you, or within your being, you will sense your awareness radiating outwards. We call this source of awareness your calm centre.

When I write of being aware, I am referring to an all-over *feeling* or *knowledge* of awareness, not the thought of it.

Holistic You will also be aware of being spiritually, and possibly even physically, part of a much greater whole: an intrinsic, inseparable and infinite part. In this context, infinite and eternal mean the same.

NOW In the state of Deep Calm you are aware only of the moment; you are not tied to the past or anxious about the future, and you have no awareness of either time or space.

When you experience this, your consciousness is in the most perfect state possible.

From this state of pure awareness, a number of things become subtly evident to you. Central to these is the appreciation that you exist, not as a physical, emotional, dreamlike or even spiritual entity, but as a point of awareness. A dimensionless, incorporeal, eternal point of awareness.

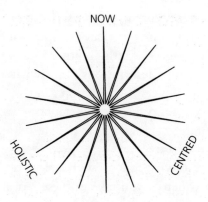

Once you realise this, you appreciate that the purpose of life is awareness itself, not what awareness provides. Without ever thinking about it again, you will know this.

There is a profound sense of comfort and wellbeing that stems from this realisation. A sense of timelessness and liberation. An experience of pure peace. This moment is the most spiritually pure you can be.

The two paths

From this moment forward, you have choice in your spiritual direction:

- you can strive to recapture and re-experience this 'awareness of awareness', extending it for longer periods, opening yourself to spiritual insight or intuition; or

- you can search for additional, more 'human' meaning.

Which is the superior path: do-it-yourself, or taking a teacher?

It depends entirely on the individual. Spiritual development is not a competition. I very much doubt whether there are more rewards on one path than another. It is the *process* that is important. It is the *process* that must be enjoyed and appreciated. It is the *process* that will make you a more spiritually evolved being.

Not the content.

The do-it-yourself route

If you choose to follow this route, you can accept responsibility for your own spiritual development from this point onwards. This is not usually a path of revelation – where one day you will suddenly realise that there is a personal God, or that Buddhism is the way you must follow. It tends to be the way of growing spiritual awareness. Where you recognise yourself and others as spiritual beings. Where you recognise the oneness of your existence. Where you give and receive good in line with the premise of doing unto others as you would have them do unto you (a philosophy common to almost all major religious movements).

How is this accomplished?

Simply through meditation. Just sit quietly, enter a state of Deep Calm, concentrate on only one thing until your mind is free of thoughts and you are aware only of awareness. The idea is to direct the efforts of the mind inwards, so that they become conscious of the mind itself. In this way the most hidden crevices of your consciousness (especially your unconscious) are exposed. This can be entertaining or illuminating.

If you choose to follow your own path – to be open to spiritual feelings and intuition – then the most reliable path is:

- meditate

- meditate

- meditate.

The more often you go to your calm centre and practise Deep Calm, the more engrained the process becomes – until you reach the stage where awareness is enhanced in your normal state. When you reach this stage, everyday activities can be transcendental in themselves. Nature takes on new meaning. Fresh air becomes intoxicating. Simple fresh foods become exotic. Love is relished, not taken for granted.

You can do this for yourself, without instruction, without guidance. When you are in a state of Deep Calm, you intuitively 'know' what needs to be known. The answers are within you. They have always been within you. You will not be able to articulate these answers – to others or for yourself – but you will be satisfied with your awareness of them.

That is one path to spiritual evolution or enlightenment.

The search for meaning

The second path is to search for additional, more 'human' meaning, whereby you discover the freedom that can only come from the study of ancient wisdoms and teachings. It involves doing all of the above – regular periods of Deep Calm where your thinking is stilled – but also includes more worldly explorations of philosophy, aesthetics and doctrine, possibly even following a guide (teacher, guru, priest, master, lama).

There is a lot to be said for choosing this path. But if you make this choice, you come right back to the beginning. What is the right philosophy, or religion, or teacher? How will you know whether one is superior to another? How will you know what is right for you?

Should you try the traditional way of Christianity, Jainism, Judaism, Buddhism or Islam? Should you consider the more esoteric religions? Maybe it's atheism, humanism, naturism, agnosticism, pantheism, supernaturalism, tarot or astrology that appeal to you.

Considering that the expectation of any of the traditional religions is that you will follow it for decades, adhering to its disciplines possibly several times a day, reshaping the course of your entire life to accommodate it, it's reasonable that you should ask, 'Is this right for me?'

How are you meant to know?

Simple: you use the complete Calm Inspiration Cycle.

1. Preparation Do your research, gather the information. If possible, do some of this preparation in a place where you are outside your normal comfort zone – this will encourage you to vary your normal thinking patterns. (It may be at this stage that you decide to consult a particular teacher or guide.)

Now you are ready to define the Consequence you seek. For example: 'What steps should I take to determine the most meaningful and fulfilling direction for my spiritual development?'

2. Start at the end Imagine yourself having accomplished the Consequence you have defined. (At first you may think that something as abstract as spiritual enlightenment is beyond your imagination. It is not; you can easily imagine it.)

Imagine what you'll look like when you have discovered this profound new direction in your life. Can you see the look of serenity on your face? Can you see how wonderful the world looks when you're in this state?

Imagine what it will sound like. Can you hear the things people say to you, the things you'll say yourself?

Now, the most exciting part of all: can you imagine what it *feels* like to have discovered this path? Can you feel how pure and invigorating it is? How spiritually fulfilled it feels?

Can you feel it?

3. Go to the centre Use the techniques from earlier in this book to ease yourself into a state of Deep Calm. Do it regularly! Do it without purpose, even though you really do have a purpose.

While in this state, don't give another thought to your Consequence. Just enjoy the peace and serenity of Deep Calm, allow your awareness to expand as it deems fit.

4. Accept the answer At the conclusion of this process, you will have thoughts. They may or may not be meaningful. Whatever they are, however poorly formulated or obscure they may seem, write them down.

5. Conscious evaluation Examine what these thoughts mean. Take your time: this interpretation may arouse some of your most creative thinking.

Now you will have one or a few suggestions. Evaluate them. Are they in accord with what you know from your research? Are they practical? Do you feel comfortable with them?

Which one do you feel most comfortable with?

6. Unconscious evaluation Assuming a suggestion has passed your conscious evaluation, it is time to evaluate it unconsciously, or subconsciously.

Ease yourself into a deeply relaxed state again. Imagine yourself using the particular approach your subconscious has suggested. If this feels comfortable, imagine yourself applying it in yet other situations.

If it doesn't feel comfortable, go back to the very first step. More research. More analysis of the available information. A different approach to defining your Consequence.

7. Integration The final stage is putting the suggestion into practice. You have the rest of your life to make it work. And, if ever the occasion arises where you feel this particular approach is not right for you, you simply repeat these seven steps.

The process of finding the right spiritual direction for you is no different from finding the right career path, the right surgeon, the right partner – the most reliable path is:

- meditate

- investigate

- meditate.

And the most reliable way of finding an inspired solution to any question you might have is the Calm Inspiration Cycle.

Choosing a guide

If you decide to be guided by someone more learned or spiritually evolved than yourself, the question is, 'Who do you turn to?' Should you listen to the one who is the most charismatic? Should you take notice of the most learned? Should you follow the one who appears to be the most enlightened? Should you believe the one who claims to be in daily contact with God?

How are you meant to choose?

Fortunately there is a simple answer.

If you have been practising Deep Calm for extended periods, if you have been enjoying it and are open to the intuitive insights that come from it, you will already be developing spiritually. So, being already on the path, knowing who is the best person to help you along that path is a much easier decision. Nevertheless, I will show you a way of making this even easier.

Simply follow the same procedure outlined for choosing a health therapist on page 277. Follow all those steps, do your homework, then follow your instincts. Not your likes or dislikes, your *instincts*.

Whichever path you take, you will be well equipped to find what you are looking for after regular use of Deep Calm or meditation. Do this for the enjoyment of the experience alone, and the spiritual side will take care of itself.

> *Finally, there is one consideration you should never lose sight of. When you approach it with a calm, open mind – without bias or expectation – spiritual awakening can be the most magical journey a human being can take. There are many phases to this journey. Once you have passed them, there is no coming back. A nostalgic part of you may want to cling to elements of your past, but there is no turning back. Once you have seen even a glimpse of how profoundly wonderful this new awakening is, you will be drawn forward on the most exciting journey imaginable.*

It may take a year. It may take 40 years. But what does it matter; you have all the time in the world.

An earthly postscript

On the way to spiritual awakening, you will discover a side benefit. A *temporal* benefit. It has been shown that those who follow spiritual practices – of any type – enjoy better mental health and emotional wellbeing than those who don't (on average).

Oh, you expected that?

Well, it can also be shown that those who follow spiritual practices enjoy better *physical* health and wellbeing as well. From a strictly scientific research perspective, this doesn't prove a great deal. There is no way of knowing whether one is the product of the other, or indeed whether certain healthy types are attracted to spiritual practices and vice versa.

But, whatever the reason, one could conclude that there is a range of sound worldly reasons why spiritual practices should be encouraged and participated in.

The big picture

One of the benefits of being able to take a holistic view of your life and your life's events is that it gives you the ability to put things into perspective.

You know from experience that if you concentrate too much on the detail of any given situation, you take on the emotions or attitudes that relate to the detail – rather than the overall situation. If you're in a crowd of beautifully behaved people but the handful beside you are argumentative and aggressive, you will probably overlook the predominantly good behaviour of the crowd and respond to the aggression of your neighbours. If you live in a nation where the economy is booming but you just got retrenched from your job, you will probably overlook the national mood and be depressed about your immediate situation. And if your partner has been a loving companion for 30 years but snapped at you over breakfast, you will probably overlook the many years and respond to the breakfast rebuke.

You can avoid these failures of perspective.

By using the practices we have been covering, you will gradually begin to develop a more holistic view of life. This happens of its own accord, and there is little you have to do to enact it. Deep Calm is especially powerful in this capacity.

But until such time as you have this perspective, here are two simple techniques to help you maintain a 'big picture' view during the difficult times.

The pattern of progress

Techniques such as the two that follow require a brief aside about the nature of progress.

In all avenues of life, the difference between progress and regress is usually a matter of perspective. Most people who have achieved anything significant in life, and who have made a difference in the world around them, will recognise this simple truism: progress is usually marked by two steps forwards and one step backwards.

If you look too closely at the detail (that is, if you're not looking at the big picture), you may be discouraged or dissuaded by that one step backwards. This is why having a powerful Consequence compensates for so many things in life – because it gives you a big-picture view of what you are trying to achieve, and so keeps the occasional setbacks in balance.

If, at any stage, you feel overwhelmed by the setbacks, you simply widen your perspective until you can recognise the pattern of progress: two steps forwards, one step back.

Go forward, look back

The purpose of this technique is to help you put today's problems into the perspective of a lifetime – not easy to do while you're enduring them today.

There are three steps.

The first is to go somewhere quiet, tell yourself you have all the time in the world, then listen to the sound of your breathing for a couple of minutes. Before you know it, you will be easing into a state of Deep Calm (because you will have done this many times before).

Second, in your mind, get a picture of yourself as you will look in 10 years' time. What will you be wearing? Where will you be living? What colour will your hair be? What will you be seeing? What are the sounds around you? Can you hear anything that's specific to where you'll be when you're 10 years older? What will you be *feeling*?

When you have an idea of how it feels to be living 10 years in the future, think about today. Now, how do you rate the problems you're enduring today? How will they have affected your life? What difference will they make? Will you even remember them?

You know how this works. In most cases, the problem will seem quite small in your overall life perspective.

The centre of the universe

Remember earlier when we worked out your position in relation to the rest of the universe? Because the universe is infinite (by definition), the edge of the universe is an infinite distance in every direction – which places you right at the centre of the universe. Let's see how we can apply that understanding in order to reduce today's problems.

Once again, this is a technique of three simple steps.

To begin with, find yourself a quiet place, tell yourself you have all the time in the world, then spend a couple of minutes listening to the sound of your breathing. Wait until you are entering a Deep Calm state. Now, close your eyes and begin to expand your (imagined) view of the world. Imagine you can see outside the room you are in. Imagine you can see past your house, into the street. Looking up now, imagine you can see above your suburb, way off into the night sky above. You can see way into space. Past the satellites, past the moon, off in the direction of the planets. Time is not an obstacle, since you have all the time in the world. Now you can see way beyond our galaxy. It's so still and quiet out there. So, so . . . *infinite*. Now turn your attention back to yourself: sitting quietly in your chair, an infinitesimal speck in an eternity of space.

When you can feel what it's like to be part of this grand spectacle, your problems will seem smaller. Once you can really feel it, they begin to diminish. You don't even have to think about them in context: when you can really feel your relativity to the rest of the universe, your problems diminish. They may even vanish altogether.

You may think this sounds a little unrealistic. What if the problem you're enduring is gigantic? Horrific, maybe. Obviously one adjustment in thinking will not remove a massive problem. However it will put it into perspective and, sometimes, you can't ask for more than that.

Calm major, calm minor

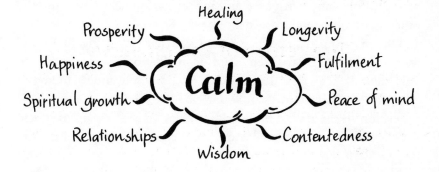

By now, you will see how Deep Calm, when combined with the Success Formula and the Calm Inspiration Cycle, enables you to achieve almost anything you set your mind to – even those things that are conventionally considered impossible.

The key is setting your mind to it.

Although some of my examples refer to the major challenges in life, the techniques need not be reserved for such matters. When you've taken time out for them a few times – and the ideal is to do this on a daily basis – you'll find they are useful for all aspects of your daily grind: planning your day's work, deciding on the paint colour for the bedroom, deciding whether to go out with someone, invest-ment decisions, job decisions, lifestyle decisions.

Better still, the more you use these techniques, the simpler they become. I have purposely explained them in great detail. In practice, especially after regular use, they become abbreviated – sometimes you can complete the Calm Inspiration Cycle, for example, in just a minute or so: very useful when you require a quick creative solution.

After a while, using these techniques becomes second nature. I use them myself – several times a day – without even being aware of the fact that this is what I'm doing. In my own experience, one of the benefits is that I can do so many more things during my working day, without confusion or the feeling that I am overloaded. I know many other people who now use these techniques in business – with the same result.

Practise Deep Calm as often as you can. Treat it as an indulgence. A special time you devote to yourself. A selfish occasion specially designed for your own peace and inner development. Then use the other techniques when you need them.

Do this regularly, and you'll find yourself becoming more and more capable. Regular Deep Calm or meditation improves the way you think. It helps you develop your wisdom and understanding of life. It helps you to understand yourself – the whole you – especially in relation to the rest of the world. It helps you to remain in touch, and to fine-tune your wellbeing, your emotions, your values and belief systems.

No other practice I know of even comes close to achieving all this.

So far, you've discovered that:

- **You have a choice of techniques that can take you to your calm centre and the experience of Deep Calm.**

- **If you take regular time out for Deep Calm, you can achieve extraordinary things.**

- **By combining this practice with the Success Formula, you can achieve anything.**

- **When you include the Calm Inspiration Cycle, you will discover the most inspired ways to achieve this.**

- **The solutions you find can transform all aspects of your life – health, longevity, success, prosperity, relationships, spiritual development . . . anything.**

9

CALM FOR THE REST OF YOUR LIFE

Although brief, this section is packed with subtle suggestions for your subconscious. For maximum effect, read it in a relaxed state (you might even choose to do it a couple of times . . .)

Now it is time to bring all the aforementioned advice and techniques into focus.

The starting point is to recognise what I believe is the greatest cause of emotional stress in the world today. It is not chemical pollution, the negativity of the media, intense competitiveness, population growth or the pressure of time. It is the attempt to preserve order.

Once, this was a peculiarly Western condition. Now it is universal. For reasons which I can only speculate about, people have become increasingly linear in their thinking. The left-brainers dominate in all aspects of our culture – media, business, politics, economics, religion, medicine, psychology, most of the sciences, music, literature and, most pernicious of all, popular television and cinema. Linear or left-brain thinking demands structure and resolution. It holds that all events in life have a beginning, a middle and an end.

In drama – or at least modern Western drama – storylines invariably follow this structure. While the more creative authors, speakers, playwrights, musicians and film-makers may try to resist this constraint, and take a non-linear approach to their work, these attempts are seldom popular. We, the consumers, demand this simple structure and resolution. Some believe this discipline was created to satisfy a deep human craving, but more likely it is cultural: we've been trained since childhood to expect our stories to unfold in a strictly linear fashion and, if they don't, we are left unsatisfied. This expectation is not so pronounced in many other cultures.

Today, our craving for order permeates all aspects of our lives. In matters of health, we think of ailments as having a beginning (disease), a middle (treatment), and therefore an end. Or birth, life and death. With environmental issues, we think of there being a beginning (hole in the ozone layer), a middle (science will find a solution), and therefore an end. No matter what aspect of life you examine, you will find this naïve expectation: a beginning, middle and resolution.

Yet, life is, of itself, disorderly. As far as we can tell, the natural 'order' is chaos. Everything we know of in nature is headed towards greater entropy (a measure of the disorder in any system). Nothing is fixed or permanent – not the galaxies, stars, the sun, the earth – everything eventually comes to an end, then is recycled. Trying to establish order in this chaos is romantic and doomed to frustration. Stress follows.

There is a better way. If you can accept that chaos *is* the natural order and that you might as well go with it, then suddenly a great weight is lifted from you. When you eliminate this expectation of order, you have the ability to be free.

One of my Zen teachers used to say, 'Expect nothing, accept everything'. There is a seductiveness to that philosophy. And if your approach to life is simply to participate and enjoy it to the fullest – as opposed to trying to modify it to suit your requirements – it is a philosophy that will serve you well.

If, however, you do want to exert more influence over your fate, this philosophy will seem overly passive. To make it work to accommodate your needs requires two simple steps.

The first is to recognise that, even though there may be no order in nature, there does seem to be at least one distinct pattern: things evolve or are created, they eventually come to an end, and then they are recycled. A pattern. A circular pattern. (Nobody knows whether this is an infinite pattern, but it will remain a pattern for the foreseeable future.)

Let's keep that pattern in mind.

The natural harmony

On one of my adventures in the East, I was introduced to the shakuhachi, the Japanese flute of the samurai tradition. (I have since produced a number of musical albums with the shakuhachi Grand Master Riley Lee. More details are on the Calm Centre's web site at www.calmcentre.com/reader; the password you'll need is 'reader'.)

Although infinitely complex in its tone and expression, the shakuhachi is among the world's simplest instruments. It has no mouthpiece as such, and consists of a single piece of bamboo with five finger holes. Not surprisingly, then, it is known for being extremely hard to play – even coaxing a single note from it can be difficult. In its purest form, the shakuhachi is an elegant illustration of the mind–body–spirit–universe continuum. To be played well, this connection must be made, and the player must become one with the music (which has been passed down from master to student over the centuries).

While marvelling at the sheer beauty of this simple instrument in the hands of a master, I was reminded of another musical experience from my childhood.

The most well-known musical instrument of the Australian Aborigines is the didgeridoo. Its design is even simpler than that of the shakuhachi: it is little more than a hollowed-out piece of wood, with no finger holes, mouthpiece or moving parts. But when played by a master, the didgeridoo produces the most hauntingly meditative sound you may ever encounter – and, in fact, it is often used in meditation and healing. (Again, more details are on the Calm Centre's web site at www.calmcentre.com/reader.)

The playing of the didgeridoo is yet another example of the mind–body–spirit–nature continuum. But where the object of the shakuhachi is to become one with the music, the object of the didgeridoo is to become one with nature. And where the shakuhachi depends on individual notes for its power, the didgeridoo depends on an endless breath. To play it, you breathe in and blow out in the one circular breathing action. You breathe in (input), control the various rhythms and textures (processing), and breathe out (output) – in one seamless process. There is no pausing for breath; the player becomes one with nature.

Recognising this connection made a lot of things fall into place for me; the experience of this flow had been with me from my very earliest days.

The Calm Continuum

One aspect of life you can always rely on is change. Those who try to prevent change are those who most suffer as a result of it.

If you want to be able to enjoy a sense of inner calm, no matter what changes are going on around you, no matter what fate or the cosmos is conspiring to throw at you, you must first of all accept the constant flow of change.

Life evolves, comes to an end, then is recycled. Energy exists, is consumed, then is converted (recycled). To every action, there is an equal and opposite reaction – as Isaac Newton's third law of motion states. Yin and Yang. What comes around, goes around. The sacred and profane. Karma. Reincarnation. You will be familiar with most of these concepts.

They all imply movement. Accepting this is the key to developing a permanent sense of inner calm. If calm is all you require, you can close the book now.

But if you want to be more assertive, and want calm and contentment *and worldly accomplishments as well*, you must do more: first, accept this flow of change, and be prepared to go along with it; then redirect it slightly so it flows in the direction you require.

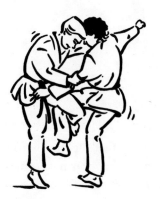

I really started to think about this second possibility when I was introduced to the martial arts. There is something very appealing about accepting all of your opponent's power and energy, then slightly redirecting it so it works to your ends. It means you expend only a minimal amount of your own energy, but gain the benefit of more than the total of your opponent's. Elegant physics, powerful dynamics.

Later, this idea of 'accepting what is, before slightly redirecting it', became a core part of my meditation training as well.

Now I recognise it as central to the concept of holism – the mind–body–spirit–universe continuum – as well as to many of the healing arts.

Accept what is, then slightly redirect it.

To make this process more memorable, I call it the Calm Continuum. It involves three parts: input, processing and output. The object is to meld all parts until they become one fluid experience – taking care to get as much satisfaction and enjoyment out of each phase – then adding a slight emphasis to them, so they move towards satisfying your particular needs.

The more seamless this cycle becomes, the more power you can exert in bringing about the kind of change you desire. In addition, the more seamless the cycle, the closer you will be to enjoying the pure experience of NOW (when you will be fully aware of the moment and not tied to the past or anxious about the future). For a human being, this is the most perfect state possible.

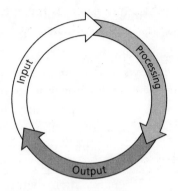

The Calm Continuum

It may take a little time and practice to get a feel for the rhythm of this, but once you have it, you will discover that you have much more control over your world than the prevailing 'chaos' would suggest. Better still, once you develop an intuitive understanding of this rhythm, you can finally let go – just relax and enjoy life.

The centre and the continuum   The most potent force in nature, the force that binds together the subatomic particles of the nucleus, comes from the centre. The most serene and satisfying place to visit during meditation is the centre. The powerful starting point for an athlete or a performer, or for any act of creation or imagination, is the centre. Balance and harmony exist when you are centred.

Being able to go to your centre – at will – is the way for you to find balance and harmony in your life, no matter what is going on around you. When you live in a chaotic, ever-changing world, it is vital that you become familiar with this ability.

You might think I am describing a very subtle experience. I am. It is more inclined to be a feeling or perception than a process. But the more you take time out with Deep Calm, with this awareness in mind, the less subtle it will seem.

All you have to do is become aware of yourself as centred, or at the centre, is be open to the 'flow' of life. Try not to force the experience; just be open to it. First feel centred; then relax and let life happen.

You already know how to do this. We have covered several techniques to help you *feel* centred (such as those on pages 87–8). This awareness of being centred is strengthened by:

- regular time out for Deep Calm;

- using additional methods for maintaining a sense of calm throughout your day.

Make a practice of calm, and you'll find it progressively easier to remain centred. Once you have an awareness of this, you can progress to taking advantage of the Calm Continuum.

The Calm Continuum means accepting that life is in a state of permanent change and, instead of trying to prevent that change or slow it down, you simply redirect it slightly so that it works in your favour. *Slight* redirection is the key.

Think of it as a spinning top. If you try to adjust a top's motion while it is spinning, you will send it awry and lose all control of it.

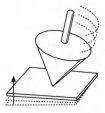

But if you tilt the surface it spins on – ever so slightly – the top will retain its momentum, but slightly change direction. So you can exert a degree of control without creating havoc.

How do you redirect it?

Your starting point is a well-thought-out Consequence that is both meaningful and important to you. This may vary from time to time. If, for example, the most important consideration you face is recovering from an illness, then your Consequence will probably relate to health in some way.

Generally, though, you will not have a major issue that you have to deal with; life itself will be the issue. In this case, it helps to have considered what your purpose in life really is. The technique for doing this is the Centenarian Test on page 239.

Then, you can subtly redirect the flow by applying the appropriate measure of Focus, Belief and Motivation, and incorporating them into the Success Formula on page 183.

The awareness of life's 'flow' is subtle. But, with time, it will become more prominent in your consciousness. Once you get a feeling for this flow or rhythm, you'll find that all aspects of your life start to develop a harmony and momentum of their own. You'll learn to make more meaningful contact with your subconscious and your intuition; in fact, for the first time, these will seem like an integral part of you rather than a hidden resource. Spiritual awareness follows. Your health becomes less of a mystery, and increased longevity becomes a real possibility. Your relationships are enhanced. Happiness is there to be experienced. The ups and downs of life can be seen clearly as ups and downs of life. Success is no longer a Quixotic dream but part of a continuum of growth.

To embrace the Calm Continuum means learning to live life using your 'peripheral vision', to listen to your intuition, to look for the truth behind the metaphor rather than trying to interpret it literally, to sometimes suspend logic and your need for proof.

And all you have to do is develop an awareness of the three elements: input, processing and output.

Input The world is full of clichés that relate to input: in the computer world, they say 'garbage in, garbage out'; in dietary circles, they say 'you are what you eat'; in social circles they say 'you are who your friends are'; in business circles they say 'pay peanuts and you get monkeys', and so on.

The lesson here is unmistakeable: if you want inspired output, you must have inspired input.

Earlier, when we were looking at the Calm Inspiration Cycle, we highlighted the most important part of the creative process – Preparation. This is where you do your homework, gather your data, do your research, study your topic and prepare your strategies. This is no different from any other undertaking in life: you must do your preparatory work first.

But that's only part of the story.

Just as important as the *content* of the input is the *quality* of the input. This applies to food (review the 80:20 formula on page 250), information, entertainment, conversation, relationships and many other areas.

Take entertainment, for example. There is a widespread belief that consuming inferior-quality television, radio and movies is a harmless activity because it 'helps you to relax'. Artistic considerations aside, this can be a dangerous belief. Regardless of how unimportant you consider the content of these inputs to be, your subconscious may not be so discerning. Seedy, depressing or negative messages always find a home – even if you are not consciously aware of the fact.

So, too, with the content of the books you read, the nature of the words you use and the quality of the food you consume.

I'm sure you get the picture. The more care and consideration you apply to the 'inputs', the better you will feel about the outputs. And, if you want to be calm for life, high-quality output is a prime requirement.

The second major area of input is not so much 'fuel sources' as thought processes. When you make a conscious effort to refine your attitudes and beliefs, so that they reflect the conscious and unconscious values you consider most important, then you make room for growth and harmony.

Sometimes this means replacing negative thought processes with positive ones (see page 100). Other times it means overcoming self-limiting beliefs with more empowering ones. Perhaps it means focusing on what you believe to be important, or motivating yourself to go the extra distance. Whatever it takes, adopting the powerful, positive ways of thinking detailed in this book will give you a level of control over your life you might previously not have believed possible.

Finally, the most significant area of input is 'receiving'. You must accept love, inspiration, compliments, prosperity, happiness, success, wellness and spiritual insight as they are offered.

For a variety of confused reasons, many of us feel compelled to reject these offerings. It is necessary to be on the lookout for this possibility in your personality. It is necessary to tell yourself – often – that you deserve success, love, prosperity, happiness. Maybe you need to adopt a little affirmation that says, 'I find myself attracting love, prosperity, happiness and success because I welcome them and deserve them'. Repeat this to yourself several times a day, write it on a card that you carry in your pocket, place it on a file that pops up on your computer each day, and soon you'll begin to accept it. Make a conscious choice to *choose* the very best quality input, then to *accept* the input you are offered, and you'll find you're well on the way to an ongoing sense of inner calm.

Processing   The next consideration is how you process this input. How can you put it to its best effect? How can you make it work for you? How can you make it fun?

In the main, there are three processing methods to consider:

(i) physical

(ii) strategic

(iii) psychic.

The physical one is elementary: eat in moderation, exercise, breathe fresh air and get good rest. Take pleasure in these, and enjoy each of them to the fullest of your abilities.

The strategic method utilises techniques like the Calm Inspiration Cycle (based on sound preparation and input) to determine the most beneficial courses of action.

And the third method, psychic or emotional, is the easiest of them all. Take time out for Deep Calm. Practise it daily. Practise it twice daily if you possibly can. Practise it for 20–30 minutes. If you find it difficult to accommodate this in your routine, at least find 30 minutes a day that you can dedicate as Self Time. This is your own special time of the day. Every day. Treat it as an indulgence. After all, you have nothing else to do in these 30 minutes but luxuriate in your own company and enjoy being yourself, with no responsibilities, no duties and no objectives. During your Self Time, avoid listening to the radio, or thinking about the work you have to do tomorrow, or worrying about how you're going to pay your phone bill. Simply put aside the time, do nothing, and allow your subconscious and autonomic nervous system do the rest.

Output   Now we get to the differentiator: your output. This is what makes the difference between mere existence and a life of consequence.

Remember the purpose of concentrating on these three areas (input, processing, output) is to highlight the fact that there is a flow to life. Recognising this enables you to vary it slightly so that it can be made to work more the way you'd like it to.

This can only be achieved when you accept the fluid nature of life, then *add* to it. In this way, you can ensure the momentum is maintained.

All of the *input* attributes you may think of as desirable – love, inspiration, compliments, prosperity, happiness, success, wellness and spiritual insight – require a corresponding output.

If you want to be loved, you must love. If you want to attract wealth, you must share wealth. If you want to be happy, you must help others to be happy. If you want to be truly successful, you must be generous with your knowledge and wisdom.

Call this reciprocity. Or fairness. Or karma. I call it the Calm Continuum. You get back what you put out – only multiplied.

And this brings us to the most important point in this book.

Spread calm

The world as we know it is coming to an end. We are poised at a point of change so extreme that we may look back on this time as a turning point in history. Perhaps you already sense this, and would not have been attracted to this book otherwise. (Then again, maybe this thought is sheer vanity.)

But there is no mistaking the change that is taking place. Issues of global economics, unemployment, the disparity of wealth between the haves and have nots, social tension, cultural instability and fraying healthcare systems are escalating by the day. The old belief that economic growth, and the discovery of new cures (for everything from AIDS to the hole in the ozone layer), will solve all life issues can no longer be entertained, because it is patently naïve. Moreover, this fact is already understood by most authorities – self-interest is what prevents them from discussing it too much.

What is the answer?

Part of the answer is to examine what constitutes national, corporate and personal success. Is it a focus on social cohesion, ecological responsibility and personal fulfilment? Or is it spiritual evolution? Is it taking into account the condensed nature of society, and finding new ways of raising the life standards of those at the bottom of the ladder? Or is our individual responsibility to succeed and excel purely in our own right? I'm sure you will enjoy wrestling with these issues.

For my part, I have shared with you a number of teachings, understandings and methods that will enable you to rise above the mundane and to accomplish virtually anything you believe is worth accomplishing in life. You now have the techniques, if not yet the skills, for making your life an event of consequence.

You also have the power to create your world as you would like it to be – making it a place of wonder, and goodness, and beauty.

But with this power comes responsibility.

And, if you want to be calm for life, your responsibility is exactly the same as mine. As I said at the beginning, my purpose is to spread calm. My purpose is to counter – just a little – some of the daily hysteria, disaster and gloom that is promoted by violent films, CNN, the evening news and the daily paper. I have chosen to do it in as wide a fashion as I possibly can.

If you want to be calm for life, you will spread calm, too.

INDEX

acid foods, 249–51

acupuncture, 13, 47, 272, 279, 284

adrenal glands, 29

adrenalin, 27–9, 187, 267

affirmation, 103, 148–9, 341

aggression, 25, 267

agoraphobia, 25

alcohol, 23, 249, 251, 264, 290

alcoholism, 25, 249

alkaline foods, 249–51

alkaline–acid ratios, 250–1, 268

allergies, 249, 267

alpha waves and states, 64–70, 117–18, 128, 130–7, 143–6, 150, 156, 221, 309–11

alternative medicine, 47

amino acids, 45, 301

anger, 24, 56, 253, 268

anorexia, 249

antibiotics, 75, 279, 284

anxiety, 24, 105–6, 253, 274, 301

aromatherapy, 143

Art of Breath, 139, 145

auditory, 110, 116, 122, 149, 151–3, 156

autonomic nervous system, 27, 342

Ayurvedic medicine, 47

backache, 249

basil, 143, 164

baths and relaxation, 19

Belief, 50–1, 184–7, 211–12, 284, 286, 300, 340

bergamot, 143, 164

beta waves and states, 64–70, 117, 128, 130, 135, 146, 150, 178, 227, 309, 311

binaural beating, 157

biofeedback, 70, 116, 118

blood pressure, 31, 102, 117, 144, 262

blood-sugar levels, 253

brain stem, 60

brainwave entrainment, 158, 234

brainwave frequencies, 64, 129, 221

brainwave patterns, 67, 70, 117, 130, 136, 158, 178

Breath of Calm, 153–5, 175, 223

Breath, Art of, 139, 145

breathing, 60

  and food, 250

  awareness of, 87, 88

  deep, 140, 153

  listening, 19, 93, 152–5, 160, 162–7, 170, 175, 190, 223, 231, 239, 269, 329–30

  slowing rate of, 13, 16, 118, 120, 138, 142, 144, 147, 154, 194, 242, 307, 310

  techniques, 141

Buddhism, 72, 123, 323, 324

bulimia, 249

caffeine, 23, 28, 236 see also coffee

Calm Centre, 33, 91, 98, 134, 149–50, 157–8, 190, 213, 283, 290, 312, 335–6

  Nine Mental Powers, 98–106

Calm Inspiration Cycle, 213–14, 225–8, 230–2, 243, 246, 277, 281, 283, 287–8, 298, 300, 303, 312, 324, 326, 331–2, 340, 342

Calm Journey, 168

Calm Walk, 159, 161

cancer, 31–2, 50, 200, 210, 249, 250–1, 265, 267, 284

carbonated drinks, 251

cedarwood, 143

Centenarian Test, 237–9, 241, 292, 339

centring, 87–8, 137, 266, 311

    techniques, 87, 89

cerebellum, 60

cerebral cortex, 60

chakras, 83, 84, 125

chamomile, 143

chemicals, 23, 31

chi, 13

Chi Kung, 12–13, 32, 139, 153, 175, 242, 272–4, 285

China, 3, 4, 11–12, 47

Chinese medicine, 47, 272, 279

cholesterol, 262

Christianity, 83, 324

chronic fatigue, 249

CLA see conjugated linoleic acid

coffee, 28, 249, 251, 264 see also caffeine

conjugated linoleic acid, 252

consciousness, 57–60

Consequence, 184–7, 190, 192, 198–9, 202–4, 211, 217, 229, 231, 236, 286–7, 289, 297–8, 300, 314, 324–6, 329, 339

    extreme, 212

    holistic, 200

    in the present, 201

    positive, 200

    specific, 199–200

    techniques, 211

    visual, 222

Consequence Montage, 204–5, 207–9, 211, 212, 286, 314

corticosteroids, 27–9

cortisol, 29, 256, 267, 271

counselling, 75, 306

creativity, 40–1, 61–2, 64–5, 70, 99, 105, 207, 211–12, 216, 225–6, 246, 298

    and holism, 78

crises, 227

dance, 124

daydreaming, 65, 133

delta waves and states, 117

delta-zzz, 67–9, 146, 310–11

dendrites, 63

deodorants, 23

depression, 15, 56, 143, 212, 249, 253, 255, 301

determination, 187, 213, 241

diabetes, 249

diaphragm, 139–40, 141, 153–4

didgeridoo, 157, 336

diet, 31, 100, 224, 248–52, 261, 263, 284, 290

    and holism, 78

dolphins, 158, 234, 316

dopamine, 267

Dreamtime, 113

drinking, 313

drugs, 284, 290, 301

electroencephalograph (EEG), 63–4, 117, 130, 178

endocrine system, 31, 256

energy, 4, 28, 198, 285

    and serenity, 12

energy, psychic, 198

enlightenment, 13, 47–8, 52, 106, 116, 183, 315–17, 319, 324

exercise, 253–4, 261, 264

    program, 30, 100

exercises, 12, 88

    centring, 137

    Deep Calm, 147

    jaw-relaxing, 135

    Step 2, 151, 180

exercises (*cont'd*)
    Step 3, 147, 159, 175, 180, 230, 242
    Tai Chi, 138
    walking, 159
expectations, 15, 171–2, 246, 289, 306, 312
    filtering, 15
eyes, closing, 132, 150

face, 206, 207
faith healing, 267
fear, 27–8, 268
    of failure, 295–6
    of success, 295–6
Featherlight Hand, 137
Floating Tongue, 135, 145, 310
Focus, 79, 163, 185–7, 211–12, 286, 296, 300, 340
focusing, 104, 123, 153, 271
folic acid, 252
food, 249, 252, 340–1
    acid, 249–51
    additives, 23
    alkaline, 249–51
    junk, 250
    preserved, 249–50
food chain, 23
frequencies
    brainwave, 64, 129, 221

gamma waves, 64
geranium, 143, 164
goals, 15, 185, 187, 190, 208, 236, 289, 300
God Spot, 134, 315
guilt, 20, 24, 91

habits, 29, 63, 103
    and your calm centre, 174
    and health, 290

and thinking, 61, 190
    changing, 63, 99–100, 312–14
    new, 142, 174
Happiness Project, 238, 302
Happy Pretence, 305
hatha yoga, 124, 136
headache, 74
healing, 45, 52, 264, 290
    and creativity, 212
    and holism, 78
    and meditation, 272, 274, 336
health services, 46
heart disease, 31, 249, 251
Heisenberg's Uncertainty Principle, 73
helper T cells, 267
herbal remedies, 13, 47, 75–76, 200, 279, 284
herbalism, 13
herpes, 29
Hindu scriptures, 16
histamines, 267
holism, 61–2, 72–9, 81, 90, 135, 216, 251, 275
homeopathy, 47, 284
hormones, 27, 117, 253, 271
hypertension, 31, 249
hypnosis, 43, 116, 128
hypnotherapy, 148
hypothalamus, 84

i (inspiration), 186, 225–6, 246
imagination, 93, 105–6, 125, 136, 140, 142, 149, 169, 212, 229
    and breathing, 140
    power of, 102
    the Calm Journey, 168
immune system, 28–32, 36, 256, 267–8, 291
    and meditation, 270–1
    and mood, 268, 270

immune system (*cont'd*)
   and stimulation, 29
   and thoughts, 267
immunoglobulin, 268
incense, 84, 143
India, 21, 47
insecticides, 23
integration, 326
interferon, 267
Iran, 47
Islam, 324
Israel, 47

Jainism, 123, 324
Japan, 11
jaw-relaxing exercises, 135
jogging, 161
Judaism, 324

Korea, 11

lactic acid, 253
lamda waves, 64
laughter, 31, 256
lavender, 19, 119, 143, 164
left brain, 60–2, 129, 202, 206, 216, 219,
   222, 227, 230, 309, 334
lemongrass, 143
Listen, 113–114, 154–5
listening, 152, 154–5, 166
loneliness, 31, 212
longevity, 71, 111, 245, 247–8, 255–6,
   262–3, 275, 332, 340
   and meditation, 262
luck, 51, 183, 256–7, 292, 299–300
lungs, 140–1, 153–4

make-up, 23
malnutrition, 249

mandala, 83, 123, 166
manic depression, 29
mantras, 16–17
martial arts, 12–13, 82, 89–90, 137, 191,
   273, 306, 337
   and breathing, 140
   and holism, 78
   and meditation, 88–9, 258
   Art of Breath, 139
massage, 119, 144, 163–5, 272
   self-, 164
meditation, 2, 78, 82, 114–15, 118
   aims of, 62
   and Art of Breath, 139
   and brainwaves, 67–9
   and Deep Calm, 117, 147, 149–50,
     261, 271, 321, 323, 327, 332
   and enlightenment, 183
   and healing, 272, 274, 279, 336
   and immune system, 270–1
   and longevity, 262, 264
   and mandala, 123
   and mantras, 16–17
   and martial arts, 88–9, 258
   and stress, 75
   and yoga, 13, 29
   approaches to, 121–5
   as therapy, 31
   centring, 88
   demystifying, 11
   postures, 155
   powers of, 32
   programs, 30
   research, 84, 112
   schools, 114, 122–4, 168
   techniques, 68, 115–17, 120, 122–5,
     141, 152, 154, 161, 175, 320
   traditions, 83, 112, 124, 126
   Zen Breathing, 153
melatonin, 267

mental health
    and holism, 78
migraine, 249
milk, 252
mind machines, 158
mindfulness, 122–4, 149
minerals, 301
mood, 143, 195, 250, 262, 268–70
    and exercise, 253
    and music, 144, 156
    disorders, 301
Motivation, 184–8, 211–12, 286, 300, 340
music, 64, 89, 102, 119, 122, 144, 156–7
    and holism, 78
    and mood, 144, 156
    relaxation, 156

naturopathy, 47
negative stresses, 31
neroli, 143, 164
nervous system, 18, 27–29, 31
    stimulation, 29
neurochemicals, 117, 143, 256, 262
neurofeedback, 70, 112, 132
New Age, 49, 78, 158
nicotine, 23, 28
Nine Mental Powers, 98–106, 149–150,
    190, 192, 202, 213, 290, 312, 317
noradrenalin, 267
NOW, 24, 89–91, 93, 95, 102, 106, 133,
    153, 201, 257, 322, 338
nutrition, 249

obesity, 249
oils, 143, 164
    essential, 143
    lavender, 19
    rose, 19
oki yoga, 136

optimism, 4, 200, 255–6, 268
orange blossom, 143, 164
osteopathy, 47

panic, 87, 213
parasympathetic nervous system, 27, 28,
    29
patchouli, 143, 164
PCR (Programmed Conditioned
    Response), 174–5
peripheral vision, 80–1, 133, 159–60, 163,
    166–7, 310, 321, 340
persistence, 241–2
pessimism, 200, 268
pesticides, 23
physiology, 133
placebos, 50, 265
pollution, 23–4, 31
posture, 136–7, 161, 170, 226
Power of Calm, 98–9, 213, 312, 317
Power of Choice, 98–9
Power of Emotion, 98, 101
Power of Focus, 98, 104
Power of Imagination, 98, 102
Power of NOW, 98, 105
Power of Repetition, 98, 102, 149
Power of Substitution, 98, 100, 150, 190,
    290, 314
Power of the Subconscious, 98, 100
Prescription for Focus Choice, 196
preventative medicine, 46
Programmed Conditioned Response
    (PCR), 174–5
psychic energy, 83, 198
psychoneuro-immunology (PNI), 267
psychotherapy, 148, 310
pulse, 13
punctuality, 24

reductionism, 71–7, 216, 251
reflexology, 144, 164

reiki, 124

relationships, 26, 306, 308, 311, 340
    and choices, 7
    attitudes, 20
    disappointments, 24
    role of, 4

relaxation, 68, 70, 120, 130, 144, 156,
    262, 304
    and stimulation, 18
    deeper levels, 182
    desirability, 19
    music, 156
    therapy, 143

remedies
    herbal, 13, 47, 75–6, 200, 279, 284
    natural, 279

repetition, 102–3, 171

research, 2, 11, 15, 32, 44–5, 47, 326, 328

restlessness, 19, 147

revelation, 315, 317–19, 323

rhythm patterns, 158

right brain, 60–2, 202, 206–7, 216, 219,
    309

rosaries, 17

rowing, 161

sadness, 24

sandalwood, 143, 164

schizophrenia, 29

scriptures, 10, 16, 317

Self Time, 173–4, 342

self-editing, 218

self-help, 103

self-massage, 164

self-perception, 61

serenity, 12, 118, 147, 325

serotonin, 267

shakuhachi, 35, 157, 335–6

shamanism, 122, 124, 157, 271

shiatsu, 124

silence, 110–11, 113, 114

sleep, 12, 33, 267

smiling, 143, 304

smoking, 28, 44, 100, 201, 256, 290, 313

somatic system, 27

sound and light machines, 158

sound entrainment, 158

speech, slowed, 142, 194, 307

spiritual awareness, 71, 119, 245, 319,
    323, 340

spiritual enlightenment, 325

spirituality
    and holism, 78

Step 1, 128, 129, 131, 146, 176

Step 2, 128, 130–1, 136, 144–7, 149, 151,
    156, 176, 261

Step 3, 128–9, 145–7, 149, 151, 159, 163,
    171, 173–6, 217–18, 229–30, 261, 287

Step 4, 129, 176–8

stimulants, 28

stimulation, 28, 64
    absence of, 19
    and immune system, 29
    and relaxation, 18

strategies see techniques

stress, 20–1, 23, 25, 29, 31, 256, 260, 301
    and beta waves, 64
    and creativity, 212
    and Deep Calm, 313
    and habits, 29, 290
    and illnesses, 31
    and immune system, 75, 267, 271
    and meditation, 75, 270
    and walking, 159
    approaches to, 23
    characteristics, 28
    chemical, 22, 31
    development, 29
    emotional, 22–3, 26, 334
    management, 18

stress (*cont'd*)

mechanical, 22

negative, 31, 262

physical, 22, 30, 87

positive, 31

responses, 29–30

symptoms, 22, 27

therapists, 28

time, 23

Strokes of Calm, 163, 165

subconscious, 20, 59, 65–7, 69–70, 101, 103, 149

power of, 100

Success Formula, 183, 199, 212, 243, 246, 277, 298, 314, 331–2, 340

sugar, 28, 249

surgery, 279, 284

swimming, 86, 161

sympathetic nervous system, 27–8, 31, 253

synchronicity, 234–5

Tai Chi, 13, 124–5, 136–7, 153, 161

exercises, 138

Taiwan, 11

Tantric malas, 17

Taoism, 72

tea, 249, 251

techniques, 5, 14, 51, 91, 152, 289, 320, 344

action, 124

affirmation, 148, 149

Art of Breath, 139

auditory, 122, 151, 156

biofeedback, 116

Breath of Calm, 153

breathing, 141

calm centre, 145

Calm Inspiration Cycle, 232, 342

cards, 202

techniques (*cont'd*)

Centenarian Test, 241, 339

centring, 84, 87, 89, 137, 144, 311, 339

cerebral, 123

choosing, 6, 171, 173, 282, 332

Consequence, 211

creativity, 70

Deep Calm, 121, 128, 159, 172, 182, 325, 328–30

healing, 124, 273

holistic, 78

hypnosis, 116

imagination, 125, 140, 151

jaw-relaxing, 135

martial arts, 13

massage, 164

meditation, 31–2, 34, 68, 112, 115–17, 120, 122, 124–5, 139, 152, 154, 168, 258, 273, 320

mindfulness, 124

Nine Mental Powers, 99–107

NOW, 257

pleasurable, 11

reductionist, 71

relaxation, 26, 262

research, 11, 15, 84

Self Time, 173–4

spreading calm, 307, 308

Step 2, 261

Step 3, 145–6, 149, 163, 171, 173–6, 229, 261, 287

Step 4, 129

traditional, 115, 116

Uplift, 137

visual, 123, 151, 166–7

wakeup, 214

walking, 161

yoga, 136, 153

theta waves and states, 64, 66–70, 113, 117, 129, 146, 221, 309, 311

third parties, 277, 280

thought, nature of, 150

Tibet, 11, 47

Tongue, Floating, 135, 145

tonsillitis, 29

Total Awareness, 162, 163

touch, 69, 79, 113, 144, 149

trance, 121

transcendence, 316

unconscious evaluation, 228, 230, 326

United States, 46, 48

Uplift, 136–7, 145, 161

Vedas, 16

Vision of Calm, 165, 167

vision, peripheral, 166–7

    widening, 163

visual, 61, 80–81, 116, 122, 149, 151

visual perspective, 81

visual techniques, 123

visualisation, 202–3, 286

vitamins, 272, 279, 284, 301

wake-up technique, 214

walking, 60, 99, 124, 159–61, 254

    and stress, 159

    breathing, 160

wellbeing, 22, 31, 33, 46, 118, 139, 147,
    247, 248, 253, 280–1, 322, 328

    and holism, 78

    sense of, 17

wellness, 31, 72, 248–9, 251, 281, 284,
    285–7, 343

whales, 158, 168, 234

willpower, 56, 57, 100–1, 131, 141

workplace, 20

worries, 20, 31, 105

    as fictions, 24

Wu Shu, 12

Yin–Yang, 83

ylang ylang, 143, 164

yoga, 124, 136, 139, 153, 175

    and meditation, 13, 29

    Art of Breath, 139

yogic state, 14, 67

yogis, 67, 178, 242

Zen, 35, 123, 257, 335

Zen Breathing Meditation, 153

Zen flute, 157

ALSO BY PAUL WILSON

INSTANT CALM

Instant Calm is packed with immediate, effective methods of relaxation. In addition, there are practical strategies for dealing with emergencies, and long-term remedies for eliminating stress, tension and negativity from your life forever.

Follow the advice in this book and you will:

- find instant relief from tension and anxiety
- cope better with trauma and everyday problems
- become more positive
- get more enjoyment out of life.

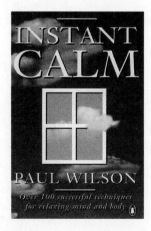

'*Paul Wilson's* Instant Calm *has captured the mood of the moment – people need serenity in their lives and they need it NOW!*'

Sydney Morning Herald